Enlightening, Adjusting
and
Savings Lives
(Fourth Edition)

20 Years of Real-Life Stories from People Who Turned to Us for Answers

(Updated with Even More New Stories)

By Dr. Paul Baker, Dr. Patrick Baker and Hundreds of Patients

www.bakerchiropractic.org

Foreword

In early 2012, we published the first edition of this book. It has become an extremely helpful tool for people who are considering our chiropractic care. We have received many compliments for publishing a book that simply allows people of all ages and all walks of life to share their stories.

We continue to receive many new testimonials from patients each month as well as updates from patients whose stories continue to develop. In 2013, we published the second and third editions of this book that incorporated all these new stories and updates. Now, we are publishing this fourth edition of the book which contains even more new stories submitted by patients.

We hope these latest real-life stories continue to inspire people and help them recognize the many benefits of our chiropractic care.

Being twin brothers, there are a lot of things in life we have endured together. When we were young boys, health problems hampered the both of us. Dr. Patrick was plagued by asthma and Dr. Paul suffered from gastrointestinal problems. With traditional medical care failing to provide a resolution and determined to help, our dad took us to a cousin who was a chiropractor in Akron, Ohio. Under his care, we were correctly diagnosed and treated with a series of chiropractic adjustments. Dr. Patrick's asthma was resolved and Dr. Paul's severe stomach pains were stopped.

From that point on, we both became fascinated and focused on becoming chiropractors and filling our lives with health. Through our high school and college years, we studied and practiced the essential elements of nutrition and exercise. We encouraged and challenged each other to adopt and incorporate the principles of health and wellness into our everyday lives. These principles are firmly engrained in who we are and why we both chose to become chiropractic physicians.

Over the past 20 years, we have been fortunate to help people with all types of pain, injury, disorder, and disease. They often times came to us out of desperation and hope. They had followed medical advice, taken prescription medications, or even undergone surgery only to realize their problem wasn't getting any better. Many times, it only got worse.

While we were introduced to chiropractic care over 35 years ago and have been practicing physicians for nearly 20 years, it still amazes us how many people either are still not aware of the vital role chiropractic care can have in someone's life or are skeptical of its effectiveness given that it does not rely on the use of pills, injections or surgery.

As you read this book, you will see how many of our patients came to us unsure or skeptical of chiropractic care and quickly realized how we could not only resolve their pain, but change the quality of their life. Our actions always speak louder than our words.

We firmly believe that everyone should reap the many benefits of chiropractic care in order to lead healthy lives enriched with wellness and filled with happiness. However, we understand that people remain skeptical. That's why we feel it's important for someone to read this book and learn why chiropractic care can help remedy many health problems.

The book doesn't contain our thoughts or our opinions. It contains the unedited words of people who had serious health problems and desperately needed answers and help.

In the pages that follow, you will see how a lot of our patients describe their first visit to one of our chiropractic clinics as "skeptical." As they tell their story, you will notice how they gained confidence in our care simply by experiencing positive results. Skepticism quickly subsides when you are open to learning and experiencing first hand.

Throughout the many stories, you will also see how patients came to us for a specific reason and the care we provided resolved not only that health condition, but many others as well.

The best testament of all to our chiropractic care is how our patients refer family members, friends and co-workers to our clinics to relieve them of their pain and health problems.

The skepticism and misunderstanding that still exist are the motivations for this book and why it is presented in this format. We didn't want the reader to study our words. We want to present the reader with the stories of people from all walks of life and have them tell their story of why they took a step towards chiropractic care for help with all sorts of pain, injuries, disorders or disease and how they came to understand the power of the human body when its full potential is unlocked by this type of care.

With knowledge and education comes logical understanding. If you understand how and why chiropractic care is effective in treating health conditions, it will allow you to see why it can be a vital part of your future and the quality of your life.

We hope the various stories contained within this book may restore hope and promise if you or a loved one is battling a health problem. We also hope it inspires you to look at chiropractic care for answers. It truly is a safe, proven and powerful form of health care.

To learn more about our chiropractic care, please visit www.bakerchiropractic.org.

To learn more about us, we invite you to visit www.doctorspaulandpatrick.com.

Yours Truly In Health and Wellness,

Dr. Paul Baker and Dr. Patrick Baker

P.S. As you read each chapter of this book, you will see some stories that have been repeated from previous chapters. Because chiropractic care addresses overall health, it is effective in resolving multiple health conditions. Therefore, if a patient was experiencing several health problems, we repeated their story for each of their health conditions.

"There is more to your spine and central nervous system than people realize. When your spine is out of alignment, it affects your body's health and functioning.

Do yourself a favor and go to Dr. Baker's office and find out what condition your spine is in and what can be done to give yourself one of the greatest benefits to your health and well-being.

Please pass this book on so others can be educated on the benefits of chiropractic care. I highly suggest you go to these doctors because I know first-hand they know what they are doing!

They will teach you and show what a lot of people aren't aware of about spinal correction."

- **Elizabeth Pinedo**

Table of Contents

1

Corrective Chiropractic Care

Many chiropractors choose to limit their practice to pain relief only. Getting a patient out of pain without using prescription drugs or surgery is very important.

At Baker Chiropractic and Wellness, we are not just focused on relieving pain. We are also concerned with providing our patients with a future life of health and wellness.

Research shows that when your spine and central nervous system are not in their proper position, they will degenerate silently. This allows organs to malfunction and become susceptible to disease. We want to make sure that doesn't happen.

We practice a type of chiropractic care known as Corrective Care Chiropractic. This form of care is aimed at keeping patients pain-free while also removing any and all interferences with the Central Nervous System. These interferences are called subluxation.

Corrective Care Chiropractic is conducted through a very specific and customized program of spinal adjustments, stretches and exercises that are unique for each patient.

The frequency of the Corrective Care Chiropractic is determined by the severity of subluxation and the position of a patient's spine. Once subluxations have been reduced and normal alignment of the spine has been restored, a patient moves into a less-frequent maintenance program to make sure they are staying subluxation-free and their spine is properly aligned.

As you read the many stories provided by our patients in this book, note how they first came to Baker Chiropractic for pain relief. Once they escaped their pain, they stayed for a life of health and wellness. That's what Corrective Chiropractic Care is all about.

Whether you are living with pain now or not, we invite and encourage you to contact us and experience the many benefits our Corrective Chiropractic Care will provide you. Your future health and quality of life depend on the decisions you make today.

Here's an example of our care from a 68 year-old female patient.

As shown in the below x-ray image, her cervical curve was restored to the ideal 43 degree curvature with Corrective Chiropractic Care at Baker Chiropractic and Wellness.

This patient's hearing was restored as a result of the corrective care.

Exp Date: 08/05/13 DOB: 01/30/1945

43°/43°

68 year old female patient. This cervical curve was restored to the ideal 45 degree curvature with corrective chiropractic care at Baker Chiropractic & Wellness. This patients hearing was restored as a result of the corrective care.

2

Not All Chiropractors Are Created Equal

Some of our patients were reluctant to come to us initially because they had tried going to other chiropractors in the past without getting the results they needed. In fact, many of the stories contained within this book are from these patients.

It's important to know that not all chiropractic physicians are the same, just like not all medical physicians are the same. If the care you were provided didn't solve your pain or health condition and didn't meet your expectations, please don't give up.

Our approach to chiropractic care and our extensive experience enables us to provide our patients with positive results that other chiropractors may not be able to deliver.

We are continually educating and training both ourselves and our staff. Decades of experience, continuing education and routine training provide our patients with the highest level of chiropractic care available. It also provides them with positive results when others fall short.

If you have tried chiropractic care in the past and didn't see the results you expected, please contact us. We are confident we will help you like we have helped so many others.

3
Acid Reflux (GERD)

"I started coming to Baker Chiropractic because I was having a lot of indigestion and pain in my middle back. In 2 months time, my indigestion is gone and I no longer have middle back pain."

- Justine

"A few months ago my infant daughter, was having severe gas pains regularly and she wasn't pooping very often. I took her into the Pediatrician when she was 4 months old and he said that it was normal for some breastfed babies to go 7-10 days between bowel movements and that she was okay. Then, when she was 5 months old, I took her to another Pediatrician since the problem had not gone away and was worse. I wanted to know what I could do to alleviate her pain. The doctor said that I should start her on regular foods (which I had put off starting because of the problem) and that the problem would most likely correct itself within the next month! So, there I was with a five-month-old child who was having horrible gas pains on a daily basis and she wanted me to wait a whole month for things to get better! I was really upset because this had already been going on for quite some time and we were at a point when neither of us could take it anymore. She was in pain and so was I because I hated to hear my baby cry when I couldn't do anything to help her. So, I asked my chiropractor, Dr. Paul Baker, if he thought he might be able to help me. He said he'd be more than happy to adjust her and he was confident he could help, so I brought her in. I was very hopeful, but didn't really know what to expect. Dr. Paul adjusted her back and neck and that night she pooped! We were thrilled because it had been so long since she had done that. I brought her in one week later and again, she pooped that night. Then she pooped the next morning and a couple more times that week. I went back each week for about 6 weeks and things just kept getting better and better. It really only took four adjustments before she was perfectly normal again. She is now a pooping machine and I couldn't be happier. She is 9 months old and as happy as can be! I can't remember the last time she had gas pains! It's a wonderful thing! I very much appreciate Dr. Paul and how great he is with my whole family and I'm grateful he was there to help me at a time when the Pediatricians didn't know what to do. It was truly an answer to our prayers."

 - **Rachel**

· · · · ·

It has been about three years; I can actually say that I enjoy my weekly visits to Dr. Baker's office. Not only has he kept me pretty well pain free, but there has been an added perk with help with my acid reflux issue. I cannot tell you in this short testimonial how many things these doctors can help people with, all without the need for medications and/or surgeries.

Kudos again to you and your staff, Dr. Baker!

-   **J. Smith**

4

ADD / ADHD and Anti-Depressants

 I first found Baker Chiropractic after injuring my back. I was standing on a patch of ice while lifting my 5 year old into her car seat. I started to slide and twisted in an odd direction to avoid dropping my daughter. I felt an odd sensation in my back when I fell then the pain started. I spent two days in bed using ice and heating pads. Nothing was helping. I had

11

always been rather skeptical chiropractics believing it was gimmicky nonsense. At this point though with 3 young children and being in such pain I became desperate. I made my appointment and met with Dr. Baker still quite skeptical. When my adjustment was over I was amazed at the relief I felt. I was able to move again. I admit I was shocked how well it worked.

My mother suffered from a lot of neck, back and joint pain. After hearing and seeing how much I was helped by my adjustment she decided to give it a try as well. Very skeptical at first she has now become a regular at Baker Chiropractics.

After being a client for a while Dr Baker told me about how chiropractic care can help ADD & ADHD. Unwilling to medicate my 5 year old for her ADD, I decided to start bringing her in for adjustments as well. She loves Dr. Baker and her adjustments. She talks about how they make her feel better.

My 88 year old grandmother lives overseas in the Netherlands. She suffers from major neck pain due to degeneration. Dr Baker has started giving her adjustments when she visits us.

After trying everything in The Netherlands from injections in the neck to deaden the nerves to major pain killers we have finally found something that helps her pain, adjustments at Baker Chiropractic.

Now nearly a year later Dr Baker is now treating 4 generations of women in my family. I am very happy I found Baker Chiropractic.

- **M. Murphy**

• • • • •

There I was last summer, coping with months of unemployment and no prospects for work. My adolescent son found refuge from the stress and uncertainty through video gaming. When he wasn't gaming, he was oppositional and agitated. He lived on soda and snacks, lost interest in sports, friends and swimming at the neighborhood pool. His posture deteriorated after spending weeks of summer vacation hunched over the laptop on the floor, addicted to an internet game.

I was busy working up resumes and cover letters, trying to score a job interview. I became concerned at how withdrawn and miserable my son was. He complained of low back and neck pain and not being able to sleep. He didn't want to attend 7th grade and exhibited mounting social and behavioral problems. He was skipping gym class, being bullied by classmates and his back pain grew increasingly worse. I did not want to have more drugs added to the ADHD medications and Anti-Depressants my son was already prescribed.

Years earlier, I had experienced positive results from chiropractic care. I wasn't sure if adolescents could benefit, but began searching for a doctor of chiropractic. I made an appointment with Dr. Paul Baker to have my son's back checked.

Dr. Baker and the staff at Baker Chiropractic transformed my son!

In less than a year, he has become positive, involved with his friends and has developed a self esteem that hasn't existed before. He no

14

longer has continuous back and neck pain; he sleeps well and looks forward to his weekly chiropractic adjustments.

Our life has been positively infused in so many ways through the comprehensive care we both receive at Baker Chiropractic.

We now focus on wellness; from what we put into our body nutritionally, to eliminating the defeatist mindset that had invaded everyday living. Our goal is to no longer use the pharmaceuticals we had relied on to manage the symptoms caused by subluxations in our spine.

I am now happily employed and my son is a successful 8th grader. Our health and well being have become an integral to a happy life and our future is so much brighter.

Our lifestyle transformation is the direct result of chiropractic care from Dr. Paul Baker and his encouraging and caring staff. If you are receptive to the power of positivity and the healing that result from a subluxation free spine, Baker Chiropractic can change your life.

- **K. Flick**

When I first came to see Dr. Baker I was lazy and got bad grades in school. I was getting into trouble all the time and not listening to my teachers. My report card was real bad and my parents were very frustrated with me. I was taking tons of medications for my ADD and ADHD. First I was on Ritalin. Then I took Concerta. I was also on Medadate and Zoloft.

Since I began treatment with Dr. Baker, I've been able to get off all my medications and actually feel like a human being again. I used to walk around feeling like I was stoned and in another world. I was depressed and flunking school. Now, I feel super and on top of the world.

I can't thank Dr. Baker enough for all his help in changing my life.

- **K. Mason**

I found out about Baker Chiropractic from another parent on my sons football team. The parent approached me and politely pointed out that he noticed my son ran awkwardly and was one of the slowest kids on the team. When Kasey was two he fell and broke his femur. He was put in a body cast for two months. After the cast came off he had to learn how to sit up, crawl and walk again. I noticed right away that something wasn't right about the way he moved and that he did not like to run. We went to different medical doctors about it several times. The answer was always the same, "He will outgrow it."

Also around the same time he broke his leg he started having asthma attacks in his sleep. It was to the point I would have to run hot steamy showers to get him to stop coughing. We also thought Kasey was a hard headed child that would not listen to anything we asked him to do. Come to find out he had so much fluid build up behind his ear drums that he could not hear us. They put tubes in his ears to drain the fluid but he continued to have ear infections at least once a month. Kasey also struggled with school work. He knew the answers to questions but was not able to process them from his mind to paper. He had a hard time blending sounds when reading simple stories.

We decided to take this parents advice to go see Dr. Baker. Come to find out Kasey's upper spine was out which was connected to his ears and his thinking process. His lower spine was also out from breaking his leg. Kasey has been seeing Dr. Baker for 2 years now and it is amazing the difference we see in him. He now loves to run hasn't had an asthma attack or an ear infection in 2 years and has brought his grades up in school from needing assistance in every subject to now being above average on most subjects. Kasey is now reading chapter books. Has a 100% in Math. He loves to play football, basketball and baseball. We are so proud of him.

Before we started taking him to see Dr. Baker, Kasey's self esteem was extremely low after everything he had been through. Now he is extremely happy, loves all sports and full of energy. We are very thankful for Dr. Baker and everything he has done for Kasey. I would and have recommended Dr. Baker to several friends. Thank you Dr. Baker.

- **The Cook Family**

5
Arthritis

After a knee replacement last summer I thought I was finally going to resume my busy life pain free. Over the last ten years arthritis had made its claim on me and resulted in two back surgeries, two foot surgeries, an ankle surgery and two knee surgeries. After years of suffering I made the decision to have a knee replacement and thought it was going to be the answer to my physical challenges. I wanted to reclaim my active lifestyle as a teacher, performer and sports enthusiast. The knee replacement itself was successful, but approximately two months after recovering from the surgery I began having horrific back and leg pain again. This time I was determined to find an answer without surgery. My son, who is studying to be a chiropractor himself, insisted that I go to a chiropractor.

So, with some hesitation and uncertainty, in January of 2011 I sought treatment with Dr. Baker. I remember my first several visits being overcome with emotion. Dr. Baker and his staff were warm and welcoming; I immediately felt they genuinely cared. They gave me hope. I was impressed with the patient education and realized how uninformed I was regarding the whole realm of chiropractic care. It was clear that treatment would take time and would require patience and a commitment on my part. After the first few treatments I could feel a difference. I improved more and more with each visit. Now, after eight months, I feel stronger and healthier than I have in years and plan to continue chiropractic care as a way of life.

So how has chiropractic care changed my life? I'm back on the golf course, riding my bike, and enjoying roller coasters again. I'm able to walk long distances and run up stairs. I'm performing on stage without pain for the first time in years. But it is in my profession as a music teacher where I have felt the most dramatic results of my treatment. I'll never forget the afternoon one of my sweet second grade boys smiled at me after we had just been dance partners in class. The innocent sincerity of his words warmed my heart and will remain etched in my memory. "I am so happy you can dance with us again, Mrs. Lewis." Thank you, Dr. Baker. Thank you for giving me my life back!

- **M. Lewis**

6

Asthma

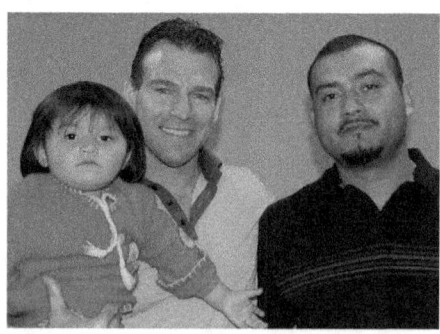 My daughter's name is Isabella Sanchez. She was born in August 2011. When she was three months old she became very sick with asthma. We were in the ER constantly because she couldn't breathe. The Doctors put her on steroids and inhalers and antibiotics. She was constantly sick.

23

After 6 months of what seemed like a hopeless and exhausting situation- my friend Angela told me that I should take her to Dr. Paul Baker, with Baker Chiropractic. When she was first examined by Dr. Paul, he told me that he has never seen a baby with so many subluxations (Subluxations are the misalignment of the spine). He told me that these subluxations were the cause of her asthma and other problems.

After a few adjustments, I could tell the difference rather quickly. She wasn't as sick and in need of as much oxygen at night. After 3 months of adjustments, she was a different girl. She was asthma free and walking. She wasn't anywhere close to walking when we started with Dr. Paul. We continue to bring her in for her weekly adjustments. We are grateful to Dr. Paul Baker for helping our little girl. She is now a happy little 18 month old toddler. We owe that to Dr. Paul!

-   **Isabella's Dad**

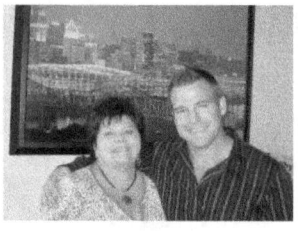

My lower back really started bothering me in February of this year (I thought I pulled something when I moved into my new house.)WRONG!

My family doctor gave me muscle relaxers, pain pills, and anti inflammatory. After a week or two with no relief, he changed the medications around and I was still receiving no relief. I was in complete agony for almost three months. A co-worker told me about Dr. Baker. I called that day, May 3, 2010 and got in that same day. After reviewing my x-rays, I found out I had many problems (not from my move) subluxation, degeneration, and pinched nerves in my lumbar. Along with all of that my hips were off!

I have to admit, the first three weeks of coming here were very difficult. I really did not know if I could continue but what kept me going were the stories that I was hearing from other patients while I was waiting to get adjusted. It is amazing how many people Doc has done wonders for.

After three weeks of coming three times a week I started having a little relief. Here it is four months later and I am so glad that I did not give up on Doc. I feel so much better, sure I have some days with a little discomfort but when that happens I just add an extra day that week to get adjusted. (I am now down to once a week!)

A couple of weeks ago I had an asthma attack. I was skeptical on where to go. It was either my asthma specialist (which was closing in 45 minutes) or go to Dr. Baker's. Danielle said, "Come here, come here!" So off to Dr. Baker's office I went. I had already used an emergency inhaler and it did not work and I started to panic which is not a good thing with asthma! While at Doc's I received EMS, roller bed, and then a massage. Massage for asthma? I said. I trusted Doc with his recommendations and after my massage with Chris and then an adjustment with Doc my lungs were totally opened! I really was amazed but I should have known he could help me, after all that's why Doc wanted to grow up and be Chiropractor. He had asthma as a child.

You will not find any other Doctor office like this one. Everyone truly is there to help everyone. They are caring, friendly, and just all around great people. Thanks to Dr. Baker, Jennifer, Danielle, Krista, Courtney, and Chris.

- **S. Mazuk**

7

Auto Accident Injuries

In June, I was involved in an auto accident. My back starting hurting shortly after, so I went to the hospital. The physician who was on call told me it was a "stiff back" and prescribed muscle relaxers and pain pills. Needless to say, they didn't work. They only made me sleep.

I came to Baker Chiropractic about three weeks after the accident. I was very skeptical at first because I believed chiropractic medicine was only a way for people to get rich who practiced it. Boy was I ever wrong!

In one week of treatment, the pain had diminished by 50%. I was able to do most of my regular activities. At the end of the third week, I was living life completely pain free. I really am very lucky that I became a patient of Baker Chiropractic.

- **R. Hall**

• • • • •

A few days after I was in an auto accident, I had excruciating pain in both my neck and head from whiplash. I was not able to turn my neck to either side; my neck and head hurt constantly. No relief was to be had. I tried numerous pain killers, but nothing helped. My mother had whiplash many years before, and only a chiropractor could help her. So I set out to find a good chiropractor. What amazing luck that I was sent by a friend to Baker Chiropractic!

From the very first adjustment, my constant headache decreased about 90%. I could now turn my neck to both sides, which previously had been impossible. Within 3 treatments, both my headaches and my neck pain stopped completely- to my great relief!

On another occasion, I had been having problems with my right shoulder. It hurt severely and I could not lift my arm over my head. No matter how much the arm hurt, I just could not move it very high. I mentioned this difficulty to Dr. Paul. Happily, he said he is a shoulder man and has helped many painful shoulders over the years. Again, I was truly lucky to have these gentlemen as my chiropractors. After the first treatment, I noticed an immense difference. My shoulder was not in constant pain any longer and I had much more mobility.

Following the Baker's program, I lost 45 pounds in a little over 2 months. Boy, do I feel better not carrying around the extra weight! I feel better than I have in years. I can move much better and more lightly.

They have given me my body back. For that, I cannot thank them enough. They truly care about each and every patient. That's a great deal to get from a health care professional.

Needless to say, they have added an immense amount to my life.

Thank you Dr. Paul and Dr. Patrick!

- **S. DeRyke**

• • • • •

I was in a car accident which left me with severe low back pain and hip pain. It was very hard and painful to walk or sit for long periods of time. I was also used to a routine of working out several times per week and could no longer do so. I have young children that were used to having their mother pick them up but I wasn't able to do that either. The stress of the accident and the pain caused a previous health condition of Crohn's Disease to flare.

After each adjustment at Baker Chiropractic, I was able to walk better, sit longer without pain and eventually return to exercising. I could once again pick up my children without any pain. Dr. Baker also helped slow down the progress of the Crohn's Disease.

- **D. Smith**

8

Back Pain

My name is Juli Gordon and I've been receiving chiropractic care from Dr. Patrick Baker for 5 weeks. What has Dr. Patrick done for me? He has done something no other orthopedist, chiropractor, spine specialist, massage therapist, physical therapist or medication could do. He has given me back my life.

For the past 2 years, pain has robbed me from living an active lifestyle. 2 years ago, at the age of 46, I was an avid marathon runner and triathlete. Over the years I've had some back, hip, and SI joint pain, but nothing that could ever keep me from enjoying a very active lifestyle. Life isn't worth living if I can't be on the go.

Due to my own stupidity, running a marathon on an injured foot, I found myself in an air cast and crutches on and off again for about 4 months. Although my foot heeled, somehow by hobbling around in a boot, I developed excruciating lower back pain that left me completely incapacitated. Now instead of running, biking and swimming, I found myself unable to do even the simplest tasks around the house without experiencing a stabbing pain in my lower back. Turning to look out a car window, picking up heavy objects, even sitting up in bed were very painful. Sleeping became an impossible feat. I could only lay on my back, literally unable to roll to either side due to pain. The stiffness and inflammation that would build up in the nighttime would leave me barely able to get out of bed and walk in the morning. I became very unsteady on stairs. With the exception of walking, my beloved daily exercise became a thing of the past. I couldn't understand how I went from being in peak physical condition to a feeble state in a matter of months. No MRI, specialist or therapist could identify and treat the invisible bullet in my back. I sadly resigned myself to the fact that I would live with chronic pain for the rest of my life.

That all changed when I met Dr. Patrick Baker. Dr. Patrick, using the Gonstead approach to chiropractic, immediately identified the problem. He was confident, even when I wasn't, that he could restore my body and eliminate my pain. After 2 years of failed attempts by other providers, in only 5 weeks, Dr. Patrick has eliminated much of my pain and allowed me to return to a normal life. Not only can I do simple things like rolling over in bed, turning in my car, and picking up heavy items, I am now able to do intense gym workouts - performing exercises I haven't been able to do for 2 years! I'm so confident that I am on the road to recovery that I am already planning for my next, most challenging marathon yet, in just 6 months.

I am totally sold on corrective chiropractic. I will continue to do my home therapy and receive consistent chiropractic care forever. If I feel this good in only 5 weeks, I can't wait to see what's in store for me 6 months from now. I'll let everyone know how I'm feeling AFTER I finish that marathon!"

- **Juli Gordon**

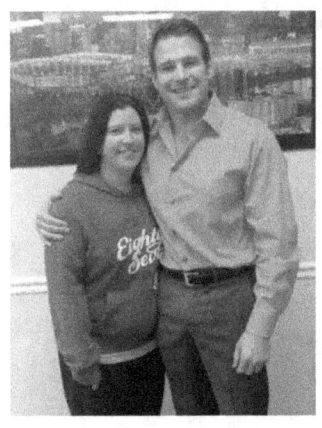 I have had back pain since I was 13 years old. I am now 35. I went to a (medical) doctor numerous times when I was young and I was always told something

different. I strained my back, I pulled a muscle, and I worked out too much. So eventually, I just stopped going to the doctor and pushed through it.

When I was young, this pain would appear and be gone within a few days, so I dealt with it. Over the years the frequency of the pain and the amount of time it took me to recover kept getting longer until December of 2012 when I hit my breaking point. I couldn't walk, stand, sleep, sit, bathe, work, or any normal things everyone does on a daily basis, without excruciating pain. On a scale from 1 to 10... I was at a 12 without moving a muscle. I landed in the ER and all they did was give me pain medications that didn't work and sent me home.

My Aunt Ann gave me the idea to call a chiropractor and I literally picked up the phone book to that section and called the first number I saw. Thankfully, the first number I dialed was Baker Chiropractic and Wellness. I started seeing Dr. Paul Baker at the Red Bank branch and eventually started seeing Dr. Patrick Baker in Fairfield. In the beginning it was very slow going. I had so many people telling me I needed to see a medical doctor and have surgery. That was the last thing I wanted. I had x-rays done and learned that my spine was curving in the wrong direction, in 2 places. And the lower curve was pinching my nerves causing sciatica pain in my left leg and foot. I was devastated, but the first thing Dr. Paul said was, "We can fix this. No surgery." I almost didn't believe him. But here I am. I'm walking, sitting, standing, and doing everything I couldn't a few months ago. I still have therapy ahead of me. You can't undo 20 years of damage in a few months.

I had a lot of people tell me that chiropractors don't help. That they are unreliable and I needed to see someone else. I am proof that that isn't true. I can say without a doubt, I probably wouldn't be standing today if it weren't for these wonderful people. I refer everyone I know to them. And I thank them all more than they will ever know.

- **Jenny Peterson**

• • • • •

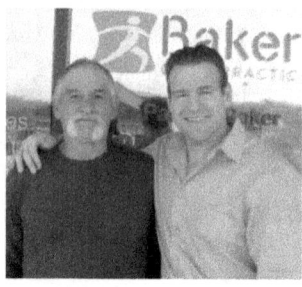

I'm a 62 year old retired concrete man. I have been doing concrete work for 40 years with 30 years of back pain. I have had two carpal tunnel surgeries and one shoulder surgery. I do not believe in taking pain pills and will not have back surgery. My dad and brother both had back surgery and it did them no good.

My daughter was seeing Dr. Baker for back pain after having two children and she asked me to try him. I did not believe in chiropractors. I decided it could not hurt so I called. Within four weeks of three times per week visits my pain was less. After eight weeks it is almost nonexistent. I went in one day on crutches with groin pain and came out without them. I can move my neck right and left further than I have ever been able to. I did not know what it was like to live pain free again.

My sex life has doubled, which was an added bonus that makes my wife very happy. I can get down on the floor and play with my grandkids again. I can shovel snow and work on restoring my 1955 Chevy, all without pain. If something does hurt I just tell Dr. Baker and he fixes me right up. I am a happy captain now.

The staff is excellent and ready to help with anything. They work with you and your insurance. I enjoy coming in for every appointment.
I cannot describe how much better I feel. If I hadn't experienced it for myself I would never have believed it. My son is now seeing Dr. Baker for his back after he had a wreck in 1998 and broke his back. He is feeling a lot of relief already and it has only been a short amount of time for him.

I would recommend Dr. Patrick Baker and Baker Chiropractic to anyone living with any kind of chronic pain.

Thank you to Dr. Baker and all his staff.

- **Harry L. Holbert Sr.**

• • • • •

To awake in the morning and go through the entire day without a conscious thought of lower back pain, could be considered a miracle for me. Having lived with chronic back pain most of my adult life; having had two major spinal surgeries (including physical therapy) and possibly facing a third, my son Kent encouraged me to try chiropractic help from Dr. Baker before I went under the knife again.

Reluctantly, I agreed and began therapy about a year and a half ago. It was slow progress in the beginning with three visits a week. Eventually, the sessions decreased to two and finally once a week. Over the past year, I have had minor set- backs (but bounce back more quickly) mostly due to excessive exercise or long distance walking. Dr. Baker discovered that my arches were breaking down and prescribed orthotics for my walking shoes. What a difference this has made!

My quality of life has so changed!! What Dr. Baker has done to enhance and improve it is beyond words. My bucket list has increased twofold: so far this year, I bought that little red convertible (makes me feel 25 years younger), traveled on my own to locations that some can only dream about and plan to do lots more before I reach 100.

Kudos to you Dr. Baker and your team of excellent caring staff!

- **J. Smith**

Update to J. Smith's Story**

Three Years Plus and Counting...

It has been about three years and one little red convertible later, I can actually say that I enjoy my weekly visits to Dr. Baker's office. Not only has he kept me pretty well pain free, but there has been an added perk with help with my acid reflux issue. I cannot tell you in this short testimonial how many things these doctors can help people with, all without the need for medications and/or surgeries.

Kudos again to you and your staff, Dr. Baker!

- **J. Smith**

• • • • •

Words are inadequate to express my deep gratitude and affection for the Baker Chiropractic Center family. I entered their doors with help walking because of the excruciating and debilitating pain in my back and leg. I met with Dr. Baker who immediately assured this blubbering mass of a broken person that he could help me. I was skeptical until talking with him, because three attempts with other professionals did nothing for me. I accepted his challenge and started treatment immediately, because I knew in my heart, that my healing had just begun.

After two weeks I felt like dancing (of course, I didn't – I wanted to, but didn't). I am better, not only because of the knowledgeable and aggressive treatment of Dr. Pat and Darren (my massage therapist) and the helpfulness and kindness of Jennifer, Courtney and Danielle, but also because everyone assured me that they would get me well. Their consistent and uplifting attitude was reassuring and healing.

Their friendliness was endearing. I feel like part of the family.

I have also met many wonderful patients, as we share our stories with each other. My continuing treatment and rehab keeps me coming back. They will not release me until I am strong enough that this will never happen again.

I have become their greatest cheerleader; spreading the word to everyone I know who has a pain anywhere, to visit them, so they too can receive the healing that I have received over the past few weeks. Help me spread the word of this wonderful team – they are the best act in town!

I've given serious consideration to dropping their business cards and pamphlets from an airplane over Cincinnati. As of this writing, my husband has not agreed to it yet. Keep looking up!

-   **J. Gilman**

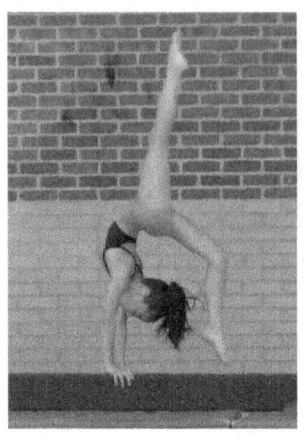

I am 10 years-old. I am a gymnast and compete for the USAG Level 5 team at Cincinnati Gymnastics Academy (CGA) in Fairfield, Ohio. I started going to Doc (Patrick) Baker because I hurt my back and when I did certain skills, like my tap swings on bars or my back walkover, my lower back would hurt. My mom said that with all of the tumbling and swinging that I do during gymnastics sometimes my body needs help to get better and stay healthy.

I went to a different doctor and his help only lasted for a little while. I liked going to Doc Baker's office right away, because everyone is so nice and I get to see Ms. Krista too! After about three weeks of seeing everyone at Baker Chiropractic my back wasn't hurting nearly as bad as it was before. Every now and then it still hurt to do my back walkover though and I would go see Doc and it would feel better right away. After another couple of weeks of seeing Doc Baker I was completely **pain free**! He even took care of my foot when that started hurting!

My back doesn't hurt at all anymore but I still love going to see everyone at Doc Baker's office and getting my treatments and adjustments. What I think is really funny, is that a lot of parents and gymnasts from CGA go and see Doc Baker now. He makes all of us feel better!

- **A. Nguyen-Storer**

• • • • •

I had so many problems with back and neck that I thought there was no different feeling except hurting and aching.

I had real bad headaches and my asthma was also bad. I felt tired and had no energy.

Today, I feel like chiropractic care should be mandatory for everyone! I never knew how much difference an adjustment could make in the way I feel. I feel like a brand new woman.

Since I have been going to Dr. Paul, my headaches, back aches and other problems have disappeared. In my opinion, Dr. Paul is the best doctor around. He is caring; he explains everything before he does it.

If anyone is hurting, they should go see Dr. Paul because he can make them feel better. If he can't, he will tell them who can.

Thank you for everything. You are the best.

-   **K. Bird**

• • • • •

I started seeing Dr. Paul in December 2009

 after I had been experiencing chronic lower-back pain. It wasn't to the point of being debilitating but I knew it wouldn't correct itself and it was affecting my ability to run. Within a couple of weeks of therapy I was running pain-free for the first time in 14 years!

Amazed by the results I wondered if Dr. Paul could help our oldest son, Aidan, who was born with a foot deformity called metatarsus adductus. The foot specialist's plan was to put our energetic, then-3-year-old, son in a cast for 6 weeks with physical therapy to follow. We didn't want him to go through that so we thought we'd see what Dr. Paul could do. Using massage therapy and chiropractic adjustments, Aidan's foot made drastic improvement.

My wife, Carrie, also started seeing Dr. Paul for her ailments and she experienced pain relief as well. During her pregnancy with our third son, she visited Dr. Paul, which helped with discomfort she was experiencing.

Our middle son, Harrison, was getting sick quite often and the adjustments Dr. Paul performed helped his immune system.

We really appreciate the professionalism Dr. Paul and his quality staff provide while also giving each patient that personal touch. Our boys are always excited to see the Baker Chiropractic staff make themselves right at home! We feel like a part of Baker Chiropractic family and because of this, we have encouraged our friends and family members to see him.

We're so grateful for what Dr. Paul's and his staff's knowledge and expertise have been able to do for our family. Thank you so much!

- **A. Kasel and Family**

• • • • •

I was having low back pain and migraine headaches. I was on prescription medicine for the headaches. My back bothered me often and kept me in bed for a few days at a time.

Now I feel great thanks to Dr. Paul and Dr. Patrick Baker. I'm no longer on prescription medications for my migraines because I rarely have them anymore.

As for my lower back, it feels great too!

They are the best chiropractors and I would recommend them to anyone. Their staff makes you feel like family instead of a patient. Thank you for everything!

- **P. Bryant**

• • • • •

 My name is Karen Tribby and I came to Baker Chiropractic because I was having trouble with my back and trouble walking.

I have been diagnosed with osteopina; complications from having scoliosis and TMJ in my left upper jawbone.

I went to see Dr. Patrick Baker because I noticed that he helped my co-worker, Craig Boykin with his back and walking. Craig has cerebral palsy and he has trouble with his arm being paralyzed and joints that just do not move as they should. I thought if he could help Craig, then maybe I had a chance for help.

50

I have been to three doctors, in the past for other medical problems and none would help including my back problems. It is very frustrating for me because when you have a serious medical problem and you hear the words, "no help", it is hard to keep you faith in doctors and people, in general. To add to my problems, I have a ventro-jugular shunt that is in my skull and I was not sure if Dr. Baker had ever heard of or worked with this type of medical procedure. I was born with hydrocephalus and this is why I have the shunt.

When I first met Dr. Patrick Baker and his staff, I noticed that they are very positive people and are committed to helping their patience's live a normal and healthy life.

I began my road to a healthier life with Baker Chiropractic in October, 2011. It has been one year now and I have had amazing results with movement returned to my back, legs, neck and shoulders. I did not realize that these areas were being affected by my back. I will continue my road to a healthier life with Baker Chiropractic as the years come. I want to live my elderly years being healthy and very active.

Thank you very much to Dr. Patrick Baker and his staff, may you continue to keep doing what you do and help people live a much healthier lifestyle.

-   **K. Tribby**

• • • • •

I've wanted to write my testimony since coming to Dr. Patrick Baker. I just didn't know where to start, so I'll start at the beginning. Over 35 years ago I injured my lower back at home. I went to a chiropractor (not to this one) for a brief time with no relief. Then I started working at an orthopedic office where I have been for 21 years. One of the doctors there over the years has sent me for epidural injections, nerve blocks, physical therapy, etc. only getting

52

temporary relief each time. The only thing that I stayed away from was pain medications and I am grateful for that. The last few years I have been getting worse, and even walking crooked. Every step was painful. I also had herniated 2 discs in my neck in 2005. Sometimes the pain would be so bad, I felt suicidal. I hadn't slept all night long in years. My husband started going to Dr. Baker when he herniated his low back. Shortly after, I had sciatica and Dr. Baker's office got me in that day. I could barely walk in, but only 1 hour later I walked out straight...and straighter than I had been in a long time! I knew right then I had found some hope! I was even able to fly to California to visit my sister. Before then, even a short car ride was painful. Every day is better. I'm even looking forward to resuming my hobbies, which are landscape photography and working in my yard. I would urge anyone who is in pain to not give up and come in to see Dr. Baker. He and his staff are wonderful! It is certainly worth it. Mere words are not enough. And did I forget to mention, I've been going there less than 2 months! It truly will be a Merry Christmas!!

-   **Carol Rice**

<u>Update to Carol Rice's Story</u>

I wanted to update my testimony that I had written in December. I had only been going to Dr. Baker's 6 weeks at that time. Now it has been 4 months since I started. I continue to get better with every adjustment.

I still feel like I am dreaming sometime. I didn't think I would ever get relief from the pain.

I am sleeping great, and am able to stand and cook the great meals we are learning to eat. Before, I couldn't stand very long at a time without pain.

Dr Patrick Baker and his staff really care about their patients.

He had a seminar which was very informative. He offered a 30 day challenge and he arranged for a personal trainer 2 days a week, all at no charge to us. My husband and I have been eating the menus from one of his books for 2 weeks, along with protein powder and supplements we purchased. We can both tell a big difference! Both of our blood pressures are down.

I feel so blessed to have Dr Baker and his staff in my life. I will never forget what they have done for me.

p.s. If this is a dream, please don't wake me!

God Bless.

2nd Update to Carol Rice's Story

I have been going to Dr. Patrick Baker's for 5 months now. I am currently going 2 times per week. Besides feeling better by getting maximized, I have gotten off all my meds! I got off my beta blocker, then off my cholesterol medicine. My last lab results showed everything within normal limits! Then I got off my blood pressure medicine. Since then, my blood pressure has been normal and a little lower than it was when I was on the meds.

Besides getting my spine in alignment, I have been eating better the past 6 weeks. Drinking 1 protein shake a day, no breads, pasta, sodas, snacking or eating out.

I feel so much better and I thank God that he lead me to Dr. Baker. I am sleeping better and have a better quality of life!

Thanks to Dr. Baker and all his staff for being here when I needed them.

- **Carol Rice**

9
Bed Wetting

I wanted to give you a hearty thanks for helping Lance, my stepson, overcome his bed-wetting problem of 11 ½ years.

As you are aware, Lance was a bed-wetter 100% of the time and it was very difficult for him to cope with this problem physiologically and psychologically. He is a good athlete and very social child and yet, had to deal with the

57

problem of never being able to stay overnight at a friend's house and the problem of constantly making excuses as to why he couldn't. In addition, he always felt like something was wrong with him because he couldn't control his bladder when other children could.

But all that changed when your treatment began. First of all, Lance has immense trust and admiration for you personally. Secondly, he became fascinated with the whole treatment process and as you remember, he would ask you a great deal of questions concerning not only the treatment, but questions about the equipment and the skeletal system.

To make a long story short, today, after only a few weeks of treatment, Lance has totally conquered bed-wetting, but only with your help. He is now 100% dry and has spent the summer with his friends including at least one overnight per week. We can't thank you enough not only your professional treatment, but the positive attitude and positive responsive which you gave to our son. I would highly recommend chiropractic to anyone who is struggling with a bed-wetting problem and would be most happy to receive calls from your patients who have questions regarding our experience with solving bed-wetting.

We thank you very much for your assistance in changing Lance's life.

- **J. Adams**

10

Bell's Palsy

I was diagnosed with Bell's Palsy. The entire left side of my face was paralyzed. I had difficulty blinking, smiling, speaking, eating and drinking. In addition, I had a throbbing pain in the back of my neck at the base of my skull.

I was told that I may have to wait 3-6 months for my condition to improve. As a speech pathologist, I didn't think waiting was an option.

I had never really known about chiropractic care, but with the encouragement of my husband, I figured I would give it a shot. I was ready to try anything at that point!

After just two visits at Baker Chiropractic, the neck pain was completely gone and the rate of improvement in my facial movement increased tremendously. At the end of the third week, I had regained 95% of my facial movement. I am thrilled with the results.

I feel that the chiropractic treatments allowed me to heal as completely and as rapidly as possible. I can smile again!

- **M. Foster**

11

Chiari Malformation

 My 12-year-old twin girls were diagnosed with Ehlers-Danlos Syndrome (EDS) four years ago.

EDS is a group of disorders that affect connective tissues, which are tissues that support the skin, bones, blood vessels, and other organs. Defects with connective tissues cause the signs and symptoms of Ehlers-Danlos syndrome, which vary from mildly loose joints to life-threatening complications.

My girls' EDS affects their spine, legs and arms. They were having severe pain, numbness and tingling in all three areas.

Dr. Patrick Baker has been adjusting them on a regular basis and they have been using their home care kits. Their pain, numbness and tingling are decreasing.

They have been adjusted since birth. Actually, their first adjustments were at the hospital.

Shortly after birth, they were both diagnosed with Chiara Malformation, which affected their sensory and motor function. They continued with specific chiropractic adjustments and showed improvement.

The Chiara progressively got worse. So, my twins underwent decompression surgery to help improve the flow of the cerebral spinal fluid.

It's 2014 and the twins still get chiropractic adjustments. They show great benefits from having a properly aligned spine.

We will continue to receive chiropractic care for the rest of the twins' lives.

Chiropractic care has been wonderful both before and after the surgery. Many thanks to Dr. Baker and his wonderful staff!"

- **Kim Skillman**

12

Chronic Aspiration

Our son, colt, was diagnosed with chronic aspiration at the age of 1 year. Along with the chronic aspiration came multiple respiratory infections, multiple doctors, multiple different medications and many other diagnoses. By the age of 2 1/2, Colt had been under general anesthesia 8 times for tests the doctors deemed medically necessary to further treat and diagnose Colt. With each test came more questions and no solutions to his problem. No doctor has ever told us why he aspirates or why he has chronic respiratory infections. The doctors are always quick to prescribe medications that they say may or may not work. What is scary to me and my husband about the medications is the horrible side effects and the long term damage the medications cause. Our frustration and disappointment were at its peak when a friend recommended Dr. Baker. We agreed to see Dr. Baker because we thought what could it hurt.

When we came to Dr. Baker's office it was a foreign environment for us. Once I got to talk to Dr. Baker and he explained chiropractic care to me, it made sense. While I was still unsure, we allowed Dr. Baker to begin adjustments on Colt. Colt was terrified in the beginning, which was to be expected, because all he has ever been able to equate doctors with is more pain. Over time Colt has grown more confident and less terrified. In fact, now he asks when he gets to see Dr. Baker again.

Colts new confidence has been wonderful but the biggest blessing we have gotten is the significant improvement in his respiratory status. He is sleeping through the night without coughing. Since we began seeing Dr. Baker he has had 1 respiratory infection, this was the only respiratory infection that didn't require steroids or breathing treatments. He was over the infection in 5 days; typically a respiratory infection for Colt lasts 2-3 weeks at minimum. Colt is now a normal, HEALTHY 3 year old who isn't taking any prescribed medications.

Dr. Baker has given us our lives back. We are truly grateful for Dr. Baker. For the first time, since Colt's health issues began, we know we are headed for success and healing. It's an indescribable feeling for parents who have spent countless sleepless nights worrying and caring for a sick child. We are firm believers in chiropractic and will recommend Dr. Baker to anyone. In fact, our other 2 children and I have started seeing Dr. Baker. We are thankful that

God put Dr. Baker in our lives.

- **The Hamilton Family**

13
Chronic Pain

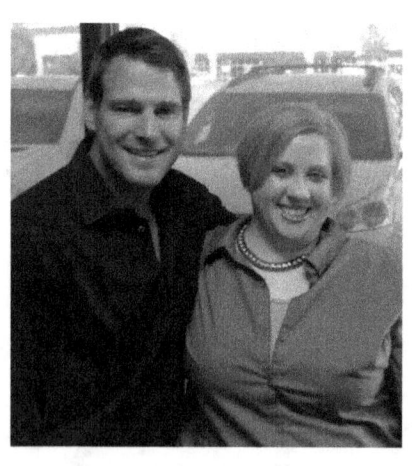

Bob Marley said it best when he said this quote: "Open your eyes and look within. Are you satisfied with the life you're living?"

Before coming to Baker Chiropractic and Wellness, I was not satisfied. I was miserable and I had no life. To be 27 years old and in constant pain robbed me of any joy that life had to offer me. I was taking a high dosage of pain medications daily just to take the edge off, but it never lasted. The pain just kept getting worse. I had been to 3 different chiropractors before with little success. I had since become skeptical that chiropractic could help me.

Within the first month, I definitely noticed a difference and now 4 months later I feel like a new person. I have more energy; I stand taller, and feel better. Most importantly though I cannot stop smiling because by getting adjusted regularly by Dr. Patrick and Dr. Paul, they have given me a priceless gift. They have given me my life back, something I thought would never happen.

I have been given a new chance to live my life the way I have always dreamed I could live it. I am seeing the dreams that I thought once were dead coming back to life because my adjustments make me feel so good. I am reaching for the stars and with continuing my adjustments, I have a feeling I will capture many stars.

Thank you Dr. Patrick and Dr. Paul for changing my life and enabling me to achieve what I once thought I could never achieve.

- Jamie Salyer

14
Colic

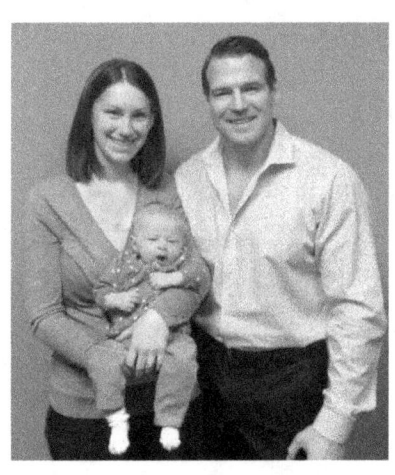

Sadie was born on Thanksgiving 2013 at 37 weeks. Almost immediately after bringing her home she began grunting, straining, bearing down and would turn bright red to have a bowel movement. She would do this several hours before having a bowl movement.

My husband and I would lay her on her back, bring her knees to her chest, give her tummy massage, warm baths, and even tried anal stimulation. Most of the time, this would not help. She started having difficulty eating and even sleeping, about an hour at time. She would wake up herself up straining.

We brought her to Dr. Patrick Baker at about 4 weeks old. After we came home, she had 2 bowl movements within an hour, and slept a consistent 4 hours that night!

Sadie is now 9 weeks old, she is now having normal bowl movements every morning without straining and waking herself up. The best part is she has started sleeping 6-7 hours at a time!

Mom and Dad are finally rested! Thank you Dr. Baker.

Emily Leimeister

My baby girl, Ellie, was born March 28, 2013, three weeks early. The first month she was having gas pains and not pooping and spitting up constantly. I took her to the Pediatrician and he said that she could go a full month without pooping, which to anyone doesn't seem logical. He said since she was early that her Sphincter needs to loosen up and that takes time. He said that he was going to put her on medicine for Acid Reflux, which I said no, as Ellie was only one month old. I immediately took her to Dr. Patrick Baker and told him the issue and he immediately said he could help with a smile on his face.

He adjusted her neck and back on a Monday afternoon. From Monday to Wednesday (the next time we saw him) she had pooped eight times and her spitting up had decreased which means Happy Mommy and Daddy.

For the first few months of her life, she saw Dr. Patrick Baker almost three times a week. Now, she goes every few weeks and is the happiest baby. I get compliments all the time for her being so happy and I always say it's because of chiropractic care. She has been sleeping through the night since she has been six weeks old, again, because of her adjustments.

A month ago, Ellie had a temperature for a few days and nothing I done would relieve it. She wouldn't sleep or eat. The Pediatrician said that she had a virus and really couldn't help. I called and talked to Dr. Brock and he came in on a Sunday to adjust her. Her fever was gone by that evening and we all got some sleep. I can't thank him enough for taking the time to come in on a weekend to help my little girl.

In closing, when we go to the office, Ellie immediately hears Dr. Patrick's or Dr. Brock's voice and smiles and giggles. She loves it there.

I just want to thank Dr. Patrick Baker, Dr. Brock, their staff and their families for the help and relief they have given my family.

- Megan Nichting

A few months ago my infant daughter, was having severe gas pains regularly and she wasn't pooping very often. I took her into the Pediatrician when she was 4 months old and he said that it was normal for some breastfed babies to go 7-10 days between bowel movements and that she was okay. Then, when she was 5 months old, I took her to another Pediatrician since the problem had not gone away and was worse. I wanted to know what I could do to alleviate her pain. The doctor said that I should start her on regular foods (which I had put off starting because of the problem) and that the problem would most likely correct itself within the next month! So, there I was with a five-month-old child who was having horrible gas pains on a daily basis and she wanted me to wait a whole month for things to get better! I was really upset because this had already been going on for quite some time and we were at a point when neither of us could take it anymore. She was in pain and so was I because

I hated to hear my baby cry when I couldn't do anything to help her.

So, I asked my chiropractor, Dr. Paul Baker, if he thought he might be able to help me. He said he'd be more than happy to adjust her and he was confident he could help, so I brought her in. I was very hopeful, but didn't really know what to expect. Dr. Paul adjusted her back and neck and that night she pooped! We were thrilled because it had been so long since she had done that. I brought her in one week later and again, she pooped that night. Then she pooped the next morning and a couple more times that week. I went back each week for about 6 weeks and things just kept getting better and better. It really only took four adjustments before she was perfectly normal again. She is now a pooping machine and I couldn't be happier. She is 9 months old and as happy as can be! I can't remember the last time she had gas pains! It's a wonderful thing! I very much appreciate Dr. Paul and how great he is with my whole family and I'm grateful he was there to help me at a time when the Pediatricians didn't know what to do. It was truly an answer to our prayers.

- **Rachel**

15
Developmental Problems in Children

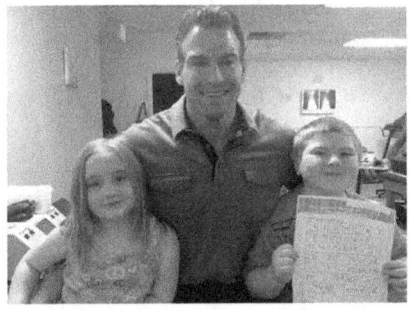

The pregnancy with my son Billy was very stressful. My labor was induced and after more than 20 hours, he was born healthy. As a baby, he was almost on schedule with all of the normal development stages, except for his speech.

78

Now 6 years old, Billy was unable to focus on anything and wasn't sleeping well. There were many days where he just wouldn't cooperate with me and wouldn't get along with his siblings. His temper was high, but I thought that was typical for little boys.

Since seeing Dr. Paul Baker for the last three weeks, I have noticed several improvements with Billy. At bedtime, he no longer takes hours to fall asleep nor does he try to nap during the day. When we are doing schoolwork, he is able to sit longer and focus on his tasks. He still needs breaks if he gets overwhelmed.

I absolutely love the changes in Billy. He was always a happy and loving little guy, but now that he is on the road to better health, he is much happier. Every day he asks me if he can see Dr. Paul and get an adjustment.

Thank you to all the staff and Dr. Paul at Baker Chiropractic and Wellness

-   **Tracy Lankford**

I found out about Baker Chiropractic from another parent on my sons football team. The parent approached me and politely pointed out he noticed my son ran awkwardly and was one of the slowest kids on the team.

When Kasey was two, he fell and broke his femur. He was put in a body cast for two months. After the cast came off he had to learn how to sit up, crawl and walk again. I noticed right away that something wasn't right about the way he moved and that he did not like to run. We went to different medical doctors about it several times. The answer was always the same, "He will outgrow it."

Around the same time he broke his leg, he started having asthma attacks in his sleep. It was to the point I would have to run hot steamy showers to get him to stop coughing.

We also thought Kasey was a hard headed child that would not listen to anything we asked him to do. Come to find out he had so much fluid build up behind his ear drums that he could not hear us. They put tubes in his ears to drain the fluid but he continued to have ear infections at least once a month. Kasey also struggled with school work. He knew the answers to questions but was not able to process them from his mind to paper. He had a hard time blending sounds when reading simple stories.

We decided to take this parent's advice and go see Dr. Baker. Come to find out Kasey's upper spine was out which was connected to his ears and his thinking process. His lower spine was also out from breaking his leg. Kasey has been seeing Dr. Baker for 2 years now and it is amazing the difference we see in him. He now loves to run, hasn't had a asthma attack or an ear infection in 2 years and has brought his grades up in school from needing assistance in every subject to now being above average on most subjects. Kasey is now reading chapter books and has a 100% in Math. He loves to play football, basketball and baseball. We are so proud of him.

Before we started taking him to see Dr. Baker, Kasey's self esteem was extremely low after everything he had been through. Now he is extremely happy, loves all sports and full of energy. We are very thankful for Dr. Baker and everything he has done for Kasey. I would and have recommended Dr. Baker to several friends. Thank you Dr. Baker!

- The Cook Family

16

Diabetic Neuropathy

 As a diabetic, I'm no stranger to pain and sickness. However, I was never prepared for the agonizing pain of diabetic neuropathy. It sneaks up on you. Starting with just a little tingle, then maybe a burning sensation. Not too bad, right? That's just how it begins. As it progresses the burning is constant, like having a match to your feet at all times until you are praying for the pain to go away. And then for the most part it does, but that's only because you've now lost all the feeling in your feet. It's like you've been walking in the snow for hours and the only sensation you can feel is pressure on your feet.

I used to consider myself to be the "Diabetic Superman". There was nothing my diabetes could do that could stop me. Neuropathy became my weakness. No matter how well adjusted or happy a person you may think you are, neuropathy will take all the joy out of your life. Want to bounce your kids on your knee? Try again, because you have daggers in your legs every time they hit your lap. It just takes all the fun out of every little thing you do, and isn't it the little things that really make us happy?

So once you realize what the problem is what do you do? If you're anything like me, you start looking for ways to "fix" the pain. I was told by every doctor I went to that there is no curing or reversing diabetic nerve damage. So what's the next step if there's no fixing it? Why narcotics of course! That's if you can find a doctor to write the prescription and don't mind being doped up all the time and developing an addiction. Not the route I wanted to take, although I did occasionally, because the pain would become unbearable. Your other alternative is "pain management".

"Pain management" is in my opinion the doctor's way of saying they can't do anything to "cure" your pain. Otherwise they would call it a "pain solution clinic". I told my doctor that I wanted any alternative to narcotics that would give me any amount of relief. You can imagine how excited I was when he told me about a new treatment called a spinal cord stimulator. It would block the signals sent by the nerves in my legs and replace them with a less painful signal. Sign me up! After more than 10 years of dealing with neuropathy this sounded like the answer to my prayers, and it was to an extent. It did indeed block the signals from my legs, but when they removed the trial stimulator I was left with excruciating pain in my back. I couldn't seem to catch a break. I didn't know if putting the actual implant in was going to leave a permanent side effect of back pain or not. Do I chance it or go on dealing with the neuropathy? To make matters worse, no doctor would admit that something was wrong with my back, despite the disc sticking out about a half inch right where my leads were put in. So after numerous MRIs, CT scans, and any other tests you can think of I felt like giving up. That's when my wife suggested I see a chiropractor. And I did.

As someone with previous experience in the medical field, I was very skeptical when I first went to see Dr. Frear at Baker Chiropractic. I don't know why? If you have heart issues you'd go to a heart doctor. So I'm not sure why I put off seeing a back doctor for back pain. Right off the bat I could tell I was going to like this place. Not only was everyone on the staff very friendly and explained the entire process to me, but how often do you see the patients happy as well? So I made my appointment, crossed my fingers and hoped he could help my back. They've done that and so much more.

After my first session, I was still sore, but by the end of the second day my back pain was completely gone. That was just the start. After every session I started to notice that I had more and more feeling in my legs and feet, something I was told would never EVER happen. So I continued to go to my appointments, and slowly but surely I'm regaining feeling in my feet. They've regained circulation and color as well.

I'm not the type of person to push any religion on anybody so I'll just leave it at this. Miracles DO happen every day. I feel like I'm proof of this. I've gone from being told that I'll never have feeling in my legs and that the lack of circulation will lead to amputation, to taking walks with my dog (and occasionally to see Dr. Brock and his staff), as well as regaining a sense of joy in my life that I never thought I would have.

I guess it pays to listen to your wife. Thank you to Dr. Brock Frear, all of his staff, and to everyone at every Baker Chiropractic office. You truly are modern day miracle workers.

-   **M. Shuhart**

17

Ear Infections

 In April of 2010 I suffered from major low back pain. So much so that I had to walk bent over to be somewhat comfortable. I was referred to Doctor Baker by a fellow co-worker. I scheduled my appointment and in I went. Little did I know this would be a life-changing event not only for me but my entire family. Besides low back pain I also suffered from dizziness, blurred vision and chronic

88

muscle fatigue and tightness. After months of prior research I secretly believed I had MS. Well, at least that's what all the symptoms on web MD told me.

After my first visit I felt immediate relief. After only a month of adjustments at three times week and lower back exercises given by Dr. Baker's staff, my episodes of blurred vision, dizziness and muscle fatigue seemed to literally disappear. Oh yeah..... I was walking tall!

Later that year my youngest son was diagnosed with his 9th ear infection. I made Dr. Baker aware of the situation and he immediately said he could help. After several conversations with my wife she felt very uncomfortable having our nine-month old adjusted. So we were referred by his pediatrician to have tubes put in his ears. After only two weeks his ear infections were back. We hated seeing our little guy in pain. My wife finally agreed to have him evaluated by Dr. Baker. That week we brought both of our sons in. After only one adjustment his ear infection was gone. Both my sons have now been seeing Dr. Baker for several months. Still no ear infections and my six year-old has excelled drastically in his sports.

Dr. Baker not only helped my entire family regain our health, he taught me how eat clean and exercise correctly. In only four short months I lost 50lbs, 5 inches off my waist and went from 33% body fat to 18%. I also was finally able to do my first pull up of my adult life. Sad but true!

Dr. Baker is not your average Doctor. He goes above and beyond and practices what he preaches. I am glad to have found his wonderful practice. I personally feel that not only have I found the BEST doctor out there but I have also gained a great friend and mentor. I recommend him to everyone I know. I have learned that traditional medicine such as painkillers and antibiotics are NOT the answer. I believe in everything this man preaches.

Don't just make one visit and hope it helps. Continue on with his health maintenance plan and you will be a new person. I know I am!! You will enjoy every visit with him and his incredible staff. Thank you again to Baker Chiropractic!

- **J. Fox**

My son had repeated ear infections. He had one set of tubes put in his ears and was scheduled to have a second set put in. He was getting ear infections every couple of months and the fluid wasn't draining from his ears.

Since coming to Baker Chiropractic, he hasn't had any more ear infections and hasn't needed to have the second set of tubes put in his ears.

- **A. Smith**

• • • • •

 We have been patients of Dr. Baker since August. Doc and his staff are helping us live happier, healthier lives, one adjustment at a time.

Tyler is a champion for Doc. He started to get adjustments after struggling with an ear infection for three continuous months with no relief from antibiotics. Each two week cycle the course of antibiotics became stronger, and our one-year-old boy was not getting better. When the pediatrician told me that we were looking at tubes I was determined to find something else. I happened to mention Ty's issue at Doc's one day; he gave me information on how chiropractic can help. We were desperate to find an alternative to surgery, so we decided to try it. After just three adjustments his ears were clear! Two weeks later he had a reoccurrence. This time we went straight to Doc. We decided to hold off on the antibiotics. And again, three adjustments later he was clear! This is such a relief to me as a mom, and our boy is as happy as can be!

Brian and Aubrey decided to begin seeing Doc in a proactive manner. Their bi-weekly adjustments keep them lined up and functioning in a healthy manner. We know that we will be healthier and happier if we can let our bodies work as they were designed. The staff treats each of us as real people, including our kids. Tyler is often in Krista's arms, and Danielle and Courtney let Aubrey color at the front. The office is a wonderful and comfortable environment that my kids enjoy. Ty even climbs on the table by himself at nineteen months!

We are blessed to have Dr. Baker and his staff as our doctor! Thank you for everything!

- **S. Dickman**

• • • • •

My husband and I are both 25 years old with a 6 month old son. I had severe lower back pain and sciatic nerve problems that seemed to never go away. While I was pregnant, my back got worse. I did not seek chiropractic care during this time, but when my son was 8 weeks old, I couldn't take the pain anymore. Dr. Baker's office was recommended to me by family and coworkers. I decided I would try their office because I knew I didn't want any pain medicine at this young of an age.

Dr. Baker sat down with my husband, son, and me taking the time to explain the problems going on with my back. During the consultation, I was given different papers talking about chiropractic care and what they can do. At this point in time, my son had been on an antibiotic for his ear infection for about 5 days (with little to no help for his fussiness/pain). I noticed on the papers I was handed that babies can be adjusted for ear infections... so I asked about that as well. Dr. Baker explained about the adjustments he could do for our little man and how it's never good to get on the "cycle of antibiotics". That night was Zeke's first adjustment. The next day, he stopped tugging at his ears. About a week later (after seeing what Doc can do), my husband was treated for his stiffness/soreness in his back and neck.

About a month into my treatment, I went to my family doctor for an ear infection. This wasn't just any normal ear infection for me. I let it go and didn't tell anyone about it until the whole side of my face hurt to physically touch. My family doctor told me the ear canal was bright red and I had a ton of fluid in my ears, and then gave me a prescription for an antibiotic. At this point in time, I was still a bit skeptical about Doc being able to help with ear infections (sorry Dr. Baker!), so I decided this would be the test. If he could help me get rid of this horrible pain/infection, I wouldn't doubt him anymore. I got adjusted right after my appointment with my family doctor. My ear/face still hurt that night, so I decided that if it still hurt the next day, I would go get the antibiotic filled and start taking it. But I didn't have to. The next morning, I woke up and the pain was almost completely gone! I was amazed! The morning after, the pain was gone. I did not have to take any antibiotics. That's when there was no doubt in my mind that Zeke not getting ear infections wasn't just coincidence. It was all about his chiropractic care!

Now, we are on maintenance care and feeling great. I don't have the pain I used to have, my husband's stiffness went away, and my son hasn't had an ear infection since (and sleeps better after being adjusted—great for us!). I can't imagine where we would be right now without the Baker Chiropractic staff. I'm sure Zeke would have had at least one set of tubes in his ears (multiple surgeries during his 6 months of life) and we would have been sore, in pain and sleep deprived at 25. We're so glad we came and got treated when we did. Thank you so much Baker staff!

-   **The Locke Family**

18

Ehlers-Danlos Syndrome (EDS)

"My 12-year-old twin girls were diagnosed with Ehlers-Danlos Syndrome (EDS) four years ago.

EDS is a group of disorders that affect connective tissues, which are tissues that support the skin, bones, blood vessels, and other organs. Defects with connective tissues cause the signs and symptoms of Ehlers-Danlos

96

syndrome, which vary from mildly loose joints to life-threatening complications.

My girls' EDS affects their spine, legs and arms. They were having severe pain, numbness and tingling in all three areas.

Dr. Patrick Baker has been adjusting them on a regular basis and they have been using their home care kits. Their pain, numbness and tingling are decreasing.

They have been adjusted since birth. Actually, their first adjustments were at the hospital. Shortly after birth, they were both diagnosed with Chiara malformation, which affected their sensory and motor function. They continued with specific chiropractic adjustments and showed improvement.

The Chiara progressively got worse. So, my twins underwent decompression surgery to help improve the flow of the cerebral spinal fluid.
It's 2014 and the twins still get chiropractic adjustments. They show great benefits from having a properly aligned spine.

We will continue to receive chiropractic care for the rest of the twins' lives.

Chiropractic care has been wonderful both before and after the surgery. Many thanks to Dr. Baker and his wonderful staff!"

- **Kim Skillman**

19

Failed Back Surgery Syndrome

 To awake in the morning and go through the entire day without a conscious thought of lower back pain, could be considered a miracle for me. Having lived with chronic back pain most of my adult life; having had two major spinal surgeries (including physical therapy) and possibly facing a third, my son

Kent encouraged me to try chiropractic help from Dr. Baker before I went under the knife again.

Reluctantly, I agreed and began therapy about a year and a half ago. It was slow progress in the beginning with three visits a week. Eventually, the sessions decreased to two and finally once a week. Over the past year, I have had minor set- backs (but bounce back more quickly) mostly due to excessive exercise or long distance walking. Dr. Baker discovered that my arches were breaking down and prescribed orthotics for my walking shoes. What a difference this has made!

My quality of life has so changed!! What Dr. Baker has done to enhance and improve it is beyond words. My bucket list has increased twofold: so far this year, I bought that little red convertible (makes me feel 25 years younger), traveled on my own to locations that some can only dream about and plan to do lots more before I reach 100.

Kudos to you Dr. Baker and your team of excellent caring staff!

-   **J. Smith**

20

Fibromyalgia

I had fibromyalgia for approximately 7 years. When I entered the office of Baker Chiropractic for the first time, I was experiencing much pain. Especially at the base of my head, down through my neck and shoulders and all the way to my lower back. I felt like every muscle in those areas was tied into thousands of tight knots. Almost any movement caused me pain and discomfort. Many other joints in my body were hurting causing me to see many doctors in the last 7 years.

I left each of the previous doctors' offices frustrated by a lack of concern and their eagerness to prescribe medications, none of which were very effective.

After 1 ½ months of chiropractic care at Baker Chiropractic, I am a changed person. I have much less pain and tightness throughout my body. I sleep considerably better at night and therefore, have much more energy during the day. Overall, from headache to muscle and joint pain and stiffness, I just physically feel better!

Emotionally, I am much better too. I am not frustrated and better positioned to cope with issues. Baker Chiropractic understands and is knowledgeable about fibromyalgia.

It's wonderful having people be excited as I am about making me feel better!

- **K. Wones**

When I came to Dr. Patrick Baker, I was dealing with fibromyalgia, spinal misalignments, arthritis, asthma and an immune system that just wasn't fighting off things like it should. I was in constant and severe pain, fatigue, breathing problems and low energy.

Dr. Baker has greatly improved my day-to-day life. With his help, my quality of life and health are so much improved. My weekly adjustments help me function better physically. I even get through flu season much better. I was usually very ill and knocked down.

- **L. Burch**

• • • • •

I was suffering with fibromyalgia. I had pain and stiffness in almost all the muscles of my body. It was worse in my neck, shoulders and lower back. I also suffered from severe headaches for at least five years.

Today, my headaches are completely gone after only 4 or 5 visits. After so many years of suffering and feeling like my head was going to explode, it's such a blessing to be pain free. I don't have to take pills to make it through a day.

-   **D. Maxwell**

• • • • •

Pain is exhausting. It becomes debilitating, it makes you irritable and it takes energy without you being aware of it. Combine pain with the side effects of cancer treatments and it becomes very difficult to find the energy and strength to handle anything.

I had multiple surgeries to treat my melanoma. As a result of these surgeries, I ended up with some nerve and muscle damage that had me in constant pain which limited my movement. I could not wear a bra due to the pain. I could not drive because I couldn't turn my head. I couldn't even lift my arms to wash my hair.

Different physicians treated me with different drugs and steroids for six months but I received minimal and short-lived relief. Not only was I disappointed in the results, I felt the source of the problem was not being addressed and my symptoms were just being treated.

Then I found Baker Chiropractic. I was skeptical at first, but I was in so much pain, it was worth a try. After two treatment sessions, a large portion of my pain was gone. I could drive again, I could sleep again and yes, I could even wear a bra again.

Dr. Baker laid out a treatment plan for me. I have been following his plan and have had a decrease in pain and an increase in motion.

- **C. Schornak**

21

Foot Pain

I just got back from the Nike World Games in Eugene, Oregon. I thought you would like to know that I ran the 100 meters in 17 seconds. I came home with six beautiful Gold Medals thanks to the wonderful treatment I received at your office for my foot.

This is the first big event I have entered since receiving your treatment. I sincerely believe had it not been for your help, I would have not been able to run at all. No other treatment I had before I came to you had helped me.

So my heartfelt thanks to the both of you, along with your wonderful staff.

- **M. Bowermaster**

22

Hand Pain and Carpal Tunnel

I had major pain and numbness in my right hand. I could not hold anything, including a fork to feed myself. I kept on dropping things and could not feel anything at all.

I feel great now. I have 100% use of my hand and no pain or numbness. I can pick up and hold anything.

Thank you to the staff and doctors at Baker Chiropractic!

T. Paragin

23
Headaches

I first started seeing Dr. Baker to help with my lower back. However, during my first consultation, I discussed with Dr. Baker my other issues I was having. Specifically, it was the constant headaches that had been plaguing me for months.

I had seen a few different doctors about my headaches and had multiple tests run and given a few different prescriptions.

Dr. Baker explained what he thought was causing my constant headaches and the success rate that they have with headaches at Baker Chiropractic and Wellness. After a few visits, my back did not bother me anymore. More importantly, my headaches where gone.

Dr Baker was able to cure what 3 doctors including a Neurologist could not.

I am a true believer in this practice and would highly recommend you talk to Dr. Baker if you have an ailment affecting you, not just back pain.

- **Robert Pape**

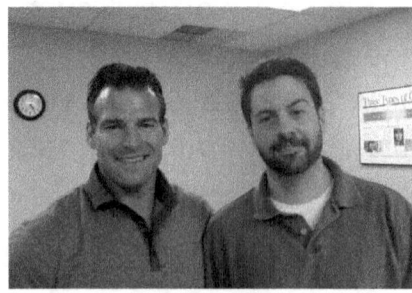

I was in a boating accident 21 years ago and suffered a fractured skull and traumatic brain

111

injury (TBI). For the last 20 years, I have been taking eight ibuprofen a day for headaches.

After the first week of adjustments by Dr. Paul Baker at Baker Chiropractic and Wellness Red Bank Clinic, **I no longer had headache issues and haven't taken an ibuprofen in over a month.**
This has been truly life changing for me. I can only imagine the damage all of that ibuprofen was doing to my liver, but what choice did I have? The pain and stress I was carrying around with me is gone and I feel great.

In addition, my entire body feels so much better. I have more range of motion now and the aches and pains (primarily in my lower back) that I had learned to live with are gone. Thanks Dr. Baker!

- **Greg Marischen**

• • • • •

I started coming to Dr. Baker due to my daily headaches that I had been having for years.

My head felt heavy and I was in constant pain. I was taking pain killers and sleeping pills prescribed by my doctor and I was also taking a minimum of 6-8 aspirins a day but nothing was helping.

Today, I am headache free. I do not have to take aspirin or any other pain relievers anymore. I am sleeping better throughout the night and don't wake up with headaches.

I feel like a new person!

- **C. Berter**

• • • • •

I suffered from migraine headaches, back pain, lack of energy and insomnia. I was taking Imitrex injections for my headaches which would provide temporary relief but they always came back.

When I came to Baker Chiropractic, the improvement started immediately. My migraines lessened drastically, I started sleeping better, my back pain stopped and my energy level improved. I have never felt better!

Had I known how good I would feel, I would have started chiropractic treatment long ago.

- **C. Combs**

• • • • •

I thought I was going to live the rest of my life in pain. I went from loving life to wanting to die. The pain that I had was slowly killing me.

I was taking so many pills on a daily basis to relieve my headaches and back pain. My family doctor told me this is all that could be done for me. I had gone from a bubbly, very active person, to someone I did not like at all.

I had all I could ever ask for in life - a husband, five children and a dog. I loved staying at home with my babies, working out almost every day and teaching kick boxing twice a week. I was truly blessed.

The family doctor that I trusted slowly took everything away from me. All I knew was pain, crying and no relationship with my family because I was in too much pain or too drugged up to do anything. I hated life!

That is until I walked into your office. I had no knowledge of chiropractic care. I didn't believe anyone could help me. I was amazed that my very first visit, I got relief. My all day, chronic pain was cut in half after my first adjustment. I will never forget that day. That was the day I started to get my life back.

My second visit to your office, I was pain free. No more pain pills. No more headaches. Being able to fall back into my old daily routine was a blessing for me.

No more screaming at my babies. No more depression. No more pills. I look in the mirror and see the person I thought was gone forever. You have healed my body and touched my heart in a way you will never know.

 I am happy again. I had forgotten what that feels like. I am amazed with the knowledge you have given me. I know more about my body and my health than I ever have. I now only have one doctor and I can never thank you enough for all you have done for me.

Thank you for not only helping me but helping my children as well. No other doctor had ever seen that one of my children had one leg longer than the other. To see them become healthier and happier children is a double blessing.

If I had one wish for those who think they have to live in pain, my wish would be for them to find you. I now know we do not have to live in pain.

Thank you for all you have done and continue to do for me.

- **T. Meyer**

• • • • •

My 6 year old son was getting headaches at least 3 times per week. Sometimes they were so bad; he would have to go into a dark room with no noise. He would also get sick to his stomach.

I took him to an allergist, and eye doctor, and a headache specialist at Children's Hospital in Cincinnati. The specialists drugged him up so much that I no longer had my calm boy. I had one that hit himself and others, tried to be a perfectionists and threw huge fits. I demanded that he be taken off the drug Amotriptoline. They reluctantly agreed but wanted to drug him with other medications.

I was searching for help and was in tears when I approached Dr. Baker. I decided to try chiropractic care and started treatment.

Today, my son only has severe headaches once or twice a year. I am so happy to have a drug free, normal boy. He is no longer violent from medications.

As a mother, I rejoice in the fact my son no longer goes through all that pain.

-   **K. Faisant**

• • • • •

When I came to Dr. Baker, I had been experiencing a headache for one week. I also had soreness in my left shoulder. I was concerned because I had been taking doctor prescribed medication for my headache and it wouldn't go away.

After my very first adjustment, my headache was gone, remarkably! I also gained significant mobility.

I'm gaining a lot of knowledge about my body and how chiropractic can really change your life.

- **M. Hughes**

24
Hearing Loss

"It was over a year ago when I noticed that I was having difficulty hearing in my right ear. The left ear was fine, but I had to turn up the volume on the TV, couldn't always hear my cell phone ringing, and was asking people to repeat themselves. I thought this was a normal aging process.

119

My husband was having issues with his neck and hips misaligned. He began going to Baker Chiropractic and Wellness for adjustments. They took x-rays and found exactly what areas needed to be adjusted. After he began his chiropractic visits, he insisted that I go and get X-rays too. I wasn't having any back or neck issues and didn't think I needed to go, but he insisted. So I went. The X-rays showed a serious problem with the L5 vertebrae in my lower back. Actually, I had 3.5 degeneration, the worse being 4.0, and Dr. Patrick Baker said it would take time to bring it back to normal, or at least to 2.5.

After I began the adjustments, I mentioned that I was having a problem hearing and had a ringing in my right ear. Dr. Patrick said he could correct the hearing by adjusting my atlas/axis near my ear. After 6 visits, one morning I woke up and heard a crackling sound as the ear opened up and I had no more ringing in my ear. I was so elated! It was unbelievable and so wonderful to hear clearly again! Imagine going to a chiropractor to get your hearing restored!

I continued my visits and Dr. Patrick said x-rays would be taken again after three months of adjustments. The x-rays were taken and much to my amazement, my whole body was in complete alignment. My neck was off by 9% and is now in perfect alignment, and L5 vertebrae in my lower back, which had a 3.5 degeneration was now 0%. I am now on a health maintenance plan and don't go as frequently as I did, however, I want to maintain good health and maximize my energy.

Overall, we feel much better now as our energy has been maximized. My husband is continuing his chiropractic treatments and wellness exercises and has shown much improvement having chronic sinus and neck problems. His hips are being realigned and straightened out to become even. We are staying faithful and are committed to follow the treatment plan that has been given to us by Dr. Baker.

We know you will enjoy going to the Baker Chiropractic and Wellness Center, as the environment is friendly, relaxed, and uplifting with a team of excellent, caring, and professional staff! We have been telling everyone about the amazing results we have had with Dr. Baker's expertise.

We hope you will visit the practice soon, as some of our friends are already receiving the same excellent care! God has richly blessed us through Baker Chiropractic. We highly recommend both Dr. Patrick Baker and Dr. Paul Baker to fix your problems as they have done for us. They are the best!"

- **Pauline & Ken Grunden**

25
Herniated Discs

I've wanted to write my testimony since coming to Dr. Patrick Baker. I just didn't know where to start, so I'll start at the beginning. Over 35 years ago I injured my lower back at home. I went to a chiropractor (not to this one) for a brief time with no relief. Then I started working at an orthopedic office where I have been for 21 years. One of the doctors there over the years has sent me for epidural injections, nerve blocks, physical therapy, etc. only getting temporary relief each time. The only thing that I stayed away from was pain medications and I am grateful for that. The last few years I have been getting worse, and even walking crooked. Every step was painful. I also had herniated 2 discs in my neck in 2005.

Sometimes the pain would be so bad, I felt suicidal. I hadn't slept all night long in years. My husband started going to Dr. Baker when he herniated his low back. Shortly after, I had sciatica and Dr. Baker's office got me in that day. I could barely walk in, but only 1 hour later I walked out straight...and straighter than I had been in a long time! I knew right then I had found some hope! I was even able to fly to California to visit my sister. Before then, even a short car ride was painful. Every day is better. I'm even looking forward to resuming my hobbies, which are landscape photography and working in my yard. I would urge anyone who is in pain to not give up and come in to see Dr. Baker. He and his staff are wonderful! It is certainly worth it. Mere words are not enough.

And did I forget to mention, I've been going there less than 2 months! It truly will be a Merry Christmas!!

-   **Carol Rice**

My name is Ken Rice. I am a 62 yr old man that had never had chiropractic care.

In 2009, I had a total hip replacement which was the result of osteoarthritis. At this time I was given a prescription of Meloxican for the arthritis. Six months later I started having pain in my neck. I went to my primary care and he referred me to a spine surgeon. I was sent for a cat scan with dye. The results came back that I would need to have a procedure to put cadaver bones in my neck due to the osteoarthritis.

After praying about my situation I decided to hold off on the surgery, at which time they recommended I stay on the Meloxican. I was also on blood pressure medications and had been for quite some time.

I am a local beekeeper in Fairfield, Ohio. In the summer of 2012 it was time to extract honey. I was out on one of the farms pulling boxes off the hives that were full of honey. Each box weighs approx. 65-70 lbs. I must have turned the wrong way and a pain shot across my lower back and down my left leg. I thought I strained something and with some rest, it would be ok. The pain didn't go away. So I went to my primary care physician. They took x-rays and sent me to a neurosurgeon. He said I had a herniated disc and we would try epidural injections. I went thru a series of those with little or no results. All the time remaining in almost unbearable pain. I couldn't stand walk or lie down without the pain. I was desperate for some relief and I didn't know where to turn.

A wonderful friend that goes to our church (Geneva Lewis) begged me to go see Dr. Patrick Baker. This was approximately 2 months after I had injured my back. The day of

126

the appointment I could barely walk into the office. I was slumped over and the pain was obvious on my face. Dr. Baker's staff greeted me and took me right back and did x-rays and scanned my back. The scan showed my neck and left lower back were severe. I waited in the doctor's and the Dr. walked in and said, "Mr. Rice, we are going to help you."

They had me hang over a machine as long as I could. He adjusted me and when I got up off that table I was standing straight and my pain was decreased by 40%. I could not believe what one visit did for my pain. With every visit to Dr. Patrick Baker's office, my back continued to improve until I was pain free!

We are still working on my neck, which was more severe than my back. I have so much confidence in Dr. Baker and his amazing staff, that I know we will get my neck pain free also.

My wife Carol and I took a 30 day challenge that the Baker Chiropractic clinic offered. It was literally a life changing experience for us. We were to use recipes from the Maximized Living nutritional plans, a book offered at Dr. Patrick Baker's office. We weighed in on a machine that told your weight, body fat percentage, and muscle mass. After the weigh in, we started our 30 day challenge. The recipes in the book I will have to say are absolutely delicious. We started every morning with a protein shake which was a scoop of Maximized Living Protein powder. That is added to 1 cup of almond milk. To that I would add fresh Kale, fresh strawberries, fresh pineapple, a few almonds. The book is a wealth of knowledge for nutritional values on various things. For example, you would need to eat 20 bowls of oatmeal to equal the nutritional value of 1 bowl of Kale. I put the fresh kale in the protein shake and when you blend it up you don't even taste the kale. After a couple weeks we realized this was a life style change we could live with. We both work, so what makes it nice is any of the recipes can be done in 20 minutes or less. The recipes literally explode with flavor. After 30 days we weighed in. I lost 14.2 lbs. and reduced my body fat by 2.8%. My wife did even better reducing her body fat by 3.6%.

An added amazing fact is that both my wife and I are off all prescription medications including blood pressure, arthritis meds, acid reflux meds and cholesterol meds. Just as a side note. The acid reflux was caused by the extended use of the arthritis med.

It is now 6 1/2 weeks and I am down 20 lbs. and my wife Carol is doing as well. We monitor our blood pressure every morning just to keep tabs. So far both are at or slightly below normal with no medications. We are at a point in our lives that we are living a much healthier life because of the total program Dr. Patrick Baker and his amazing staff offer for everyone. It's not a diet. It's keeping your spine in alignment and discovering a nutritional plan you can follow and enjoy for the rest of your life.

I thank God for directing our path to Dr. Patrick Baker and his staff. Dr. Baker and his staff truly care about your quality of life. My wife and I are living proof.

- **Ken Rice**

26

High Blood Pressure

 I came to Dr. Baker back in February 2008. I was having neck pain and my blood pressure was elevated. After doing some x-rays, we found out my neck had no curvature, my hips were off by 14 millimeters which is a lot in the chiropractic field and my back needed some adjusting.

130

Since then Dr. Baker has been able to eliminate my neck pain and reduce my blood pressure to a normal level. I'm scheduled to have follow-up x-rays in September when I go to a monthly maintenance schedule. I'm sure my neck and spine will be greatly improved thanks to Dr. Baker.

I also want to comment on Dr. Baker's staff. Jennifer, Courtney, and Danielle are some of the nicest people you will ever meet. They definitely make you feel like you're at home when you're in the office. They are always willing to help you and answer any questions that you may have. I wish more doctors' offices were like Dr. Baker's office.

- **C. Weber**

27
High Cholesterol

 I have been a patient of Dr. Paul Baker's since June 2010. I started treatment at Dr. Paul's Red Bank facility for low back pain issues. Dr. Baker is a very "holistic" doctor, concerned about the patient's entire health. I had been taking a statin for high cholesterol since April of 2010, prescribed by my cardiologist. After about 4 months, I started experiencing severe

132

pain in my hip and hand joints. Dr. Baker recommended that I stop taking the statin and try a natural supplement to treat the high cholesterol.

I began a regimen of taking EFAs – Essential Fatty Acids along with Niacin (Vitamin B). My cholesterol was tested at 259 (HDL-45, LDL-175, and Triglycerides-195). After being on the all-natural regimen for 3 months, my cholesterol dropped to 197 (HDL-82, LDL-99, Triglycerides-81). I was amazed at the increase in HDL without adding any exercise. I am expecting even better results once I increase exercise and have been on this all-natural regimen for a longer period of time. Thank you Dr. Baker!

-B. McCormick

28

Hypothyroidism

 About two years ago after my mother had been diagnosed with thyroid cancer so, I had my thyroid levels checked and found out that I had hypothyroidism.

Up to this point I was quite healthy and active and would have never thought there was anything wrong. Because of my mother's history and the fact that my numbers were still high after going on Levothyroxine, I began seeing an endocrinologist. She and I began tracking my numbers which had dropped from the original TSH of 9 down to 3.4. I still didn't have a lot of issues that many people who suffer from hypothyroidism tend to have, such as abnormal weight gain, hair loss, fatigue, and many more.

After seeing my doctor for about a year with appointments every three months and adjusting my medications, more hypothyroid related symptoms began appearing. The first problem was numbness in my hands and legs which my primary care doctor thought could be carpel tunnel. However, the endocrinologist knew the direct link that the thyroid has to the nervous system and she said that was probably the problem and we would keep an eye on it.

As time went on more and more issues with nerves and other systems began appearing, such as irregular menstrual cycles. Again we thought it was a complication of my thyroid which was causing this problem, but I went to my gynecologist to have it checked. I then had to have ultrasounds and other tests done to determine where this new set of issues was coming from which led right back to my thyroid.

It wasn't until about 8 months ago that the final issue struck which was my back. Up until this point I thought my back pain was some symptom of all the other issues that had been taking place and the battle I was having with my thyroid. Then as I was going to pick up a piece of paper off the floor my lower back went out. I could barely walk and standing for long periods of time was difficult to stay the least. After suffering from this back pain for about two weeks I decided I needed to have someone look at it because it wasn't getting better. Not wanting to have medicines and surgery as the only fix I went to see Dr. Paul Baker.

Dr. Paul informed me that my back was quite bad in many different places but that he could definitely help me but it would take some work. I also learned that when you have subluxations of the spine that it affects every part of your body. Dr. Paul and I discussed a treatment plan and how I would probably start to see a lot of my health issues start disappearing or even improve.

After six months I am glad to report that all my thyroid related symptoms are completely better. I no longer have any numbness or shooting pains in my hands or feet. Plus my numbers on my thyroid have now been in the normal range of 1.4 for about five months I couldn't' be happier. I am hoping that with continued help from Dr. Paul that I will be able keep my thyroid levels down and all the symptoms at bay.

Shelley Smith

29
Indigestion

I started coming to Baker Chiropractic because I was having a lot of indigestion and pain in my middle back.

In 2 months times, my indigestion is gone and I no longer have middle back pain.

- **Justine**

30
Infant Care

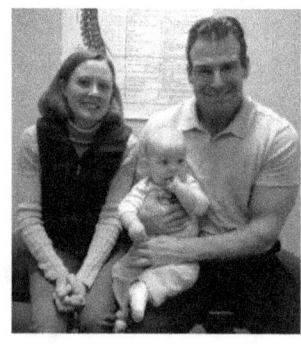 My son Jackson's birth was very traumatic. He was an emergency forceps delivery. He wasn't breathing upon birth and had to be put on a mechanical ventilator and sent to Cincinnati Children's Hospital NICU. He stayed there for a week where we were informed that an MRI

showed some damage to his brain in the frontal lobe. As a result of his birth trauma and/or the damage to his brain, Jackson's arm movements and range of motion were drastically affected. He couldn't lift his arms above his head and he carried his arms in a "bulldog" position.

In trying to address this issue, we were sent first to a physical therapist and then an occupational therapist. Neither could figure out the root of the problem with his arms. The occupational therapist actually referred us to an orthopedic surgeon and suggested that surgery might be a possibility. At that time, Jackson was 5 months old and we were still seeing the same issues with limited range of motion and abnormal posture. I decided it was time to try something else.

I researched a bit and found that the doctors at Baker Chiropractic and Wellness had the best reputation in the area with infants. I made an appointment, not sure what to expect. At our first appointment, Dr. Paul explained that Jackson's issues were probably caused by the trauma to his neck and spine when the forceps were used at birth. We started out with an intensive plan, going to see Dr. Paul three times a week. Dr. Paul was very gentle with Jackson's adjustments – Jack generally smiled and babbled the whole time!

Jack is now 7 months old and has a full range of motion after less than 2 months of Dr. Paul's care. We are very grateful to Dr. Paul and his staff for helping our son. His posture now looks very typical, and every time I see him stretch with his arms above his head, I breathe a sigh of relief!"

- B. Martin

31
Infertility

My husband and I were trying to have a baby for a long time. After months of trying and still no baby, I knew I had to try something else. I decided to start going to the chiropractor. I went in to see Dr. Baker and told him my issue. I started adjustments for one (1) month and the next month I was pregnant!

My baby girl, Ellie, was born March 28, 2013, three weeks early. The first month she was having gas pains and not pooping and spitting up constantly. I took her to the Pediatrician and he said that she could go a full month without pooping, which to anyone doesn't seem logical. He said since she was early that her Sphincter needs to loosen up and that takes time. He said that he was going to put her on medicine for Acid Reflux, which I said no, as Ellie was only one month old. I immediately took her to Dr. Patrick Baker and told him the issue and he immediately said he could help with a smile on his face.

He adjusted her neck and back on a Monday afternoon. From Monday to Wednesday (the next time we saw him) she had pooped eight times and her spitting up had decreased which means Happy Mommy and Daddy.

For the first few months of her life, she saw Dr. Patrick Baker almost three times a week. Now, she goes every few weeks and is the happiest baby. I get compliments all the time for her being so happy and I always say it's because of chiropractic care. She has been sleeping through the night since she has been six weeks old, again, because of her adjustments.

A month ago, Ellie had a temperature for a few days and nothing I done would relieve it. She wouldn't sleep or eat. The Pediatrician said that she had a virus and really couldn't help. I called and talked to Dr. Brock and he came in on a Sunday to adjust her. Her fever was gone by that evening and we all got some sleep. I can't thank him enough for taking the time to come in on a weekend to help my little girl.

In closing, when we go to the office, Ellie immediately hears Dr. Patrick's or Dr. Brock's voice and smiles and giggles. She loves it there.

I just want to thank Dr. Patrick Baker, Dr. Brock, their staff and their families for the help and relief they have given my family.

Megan Nichting

32
Insomnia

I suffered from insomnia for over 15 years. I remember the first episode when I was 12 years old like it was yesterday.

I had a pretty traumatic childhood and learned to essentially sleep with one eye open every night. It was always very limiting on my daily activities, even as a child. I always felt very tired and worn down. I never had any energy or desire to do anything and this continued into my adult life. I had to force myself to get out of bed every day due to sheer exhaustion. Any little sound or movement would wake me up at night and it sometimes took me several hours to be able to fall back to sleep.

At about age 18, I started taking over the counter sleep aids. I tried multiple brands for several months, and after awhile each one would stop working because my body adjusted to it so quickly since I needed to take them every night before bed. I eventually went to my primary doctor and later to a neurologist where I was prescribed sleeping pills for many years. We would try one and when it would stop working, I would be given a prescription for something else. This cycle went on for over 10 years. All the pills they put me on would make me feel groggy and tired the next day and it was supposed to help me feel less like that. I felt like I was in a foggy, dazed state. I began to run on auto-pilot and never had a feeling of true "rest", no matter how much sleep I would get.

I was missing a lot of work due to my lack of sleep. I wasn't able to spend any quality time with my friends or family. My husband grew very frustrated because I was frequently complaining of being tired and exhausted, and yet I was sleeping more and more. It didn't make any sense to him why I was so tired every day, and I couldn't explain it. I never had any energy or desire to do anything, no matter how much sleep the pills gave me. I had not interest in doing anything but laying around and trying to nap. We started to grow apart right under my nose, and I wasn't aware it was happening until much later.

I had been having some sever pain in my neck and left shoulder for many years, and that's what prompted my search for a chiropractor. I looked online and found Baker Chiropractic. They were less than a mile from where I worked at the time. When I called the office, I was able to get in that same evening and had my consultation and exam with Dr. Paul Baker. I got to the office and I couldn't believe how different everything was from all the multiple other doctor's offices I had been to over the years. They all actually cared about what I was going through. They didn't want me to be reliant on medication anymore. I remember leaving the office that first night telling myself not to get too excited because I had no prior success.

After making the decision that I didn't want to keep taking pills anymore, I slowly weaned off my heavy dose of prescription sleeping medications with the help of Dr. Paul. Over time, I was able to fall asleep on my own! That was something that I hadn't been able to do for so many years. It took about 4-5 months to have a good night's sleep with absolutely no pills whatsoever. I never gave up, even though there were some nights that I only slept for an hour or two. I now sleep without the aid of any sleeping medications, natural or prescription, and I am able to sleep through the entire night! I am getting deep, restful, and productive sleep. Something that I thought would never be possible. I am able to function and have so much energy and drive throughout the day, even when I have to get up before the sun comes up!

Before becoming a patient of Baker Chiropractic and Wellness, I was all around miserable. I had so many health problems, most of which I had been struggling with for over half my life. None of my many doctors before Dr. Paul Baker gave me any answers, solutions or hope. Their short-term fix was always medication. Since being under Dr. Paul's care, I have been able to get off over 10 different medications. I was taking most of those medications every day.

The staff at Baker Chiropractic was always genuinely concerned and caring, and they helped me through every situation and frustration. The many changes that I experienced were so profound that I accepted a position with Baker Chiropractic about two months into my care. Not only do I have the ability to live medication free, I have become a completely different person inside and out. I am able to share my personal experiences with our patients and help them realize what so many people don't seem to know; there is a better way!

Every day I am grateful for the opportunity to live a happy, healthy life and I could not have done it without Baker Chiropractic!

- **T. Gadrow**

33
Intercostal Neuralgia

Intercostal neuralgia is a health condition that causes pain with the intercostal nerves. These nerves are located between your ribs. Margaret came to us with pain in her upper ribs that would travel across her chest. She went to other doctors looking for answers but didn't find them. A friend told her about Dr. Patrick Baker and she came to us. Dr. Baker diagnosed

150

her pain as chronic intercostals neuralgia. Now, she is pain-free.

"The last part of February 2011 I began to have pain in my left upper ribs. The pain would travel across my chest. I thought I was having a heart attack.

I went to my primary care doctor and she said it must be from my back and sent me to a pain management clinic. This was after three x-rays, a fully body scan and one shot for pain.

After the first injection, the pain worsened and I was sent for an MRI with contrast. The doctors told me if I was not better after the third injection then I should see another doctor. So, I called my husband's doctor that did his back surgery. After another MRI, he said there was nothing wrong with my back.

After a few months of pain that was getting worse every day, a friend told me about coming to Dr. Patrick Baker. I called and was in the office in just days. When I told Dr. Baker the pain was in my ribs – not my back, he and his staff began treatment that now has me pain-free!

151

Thank you Dr. Baker and Staff."

- **Margaret Kitts**

34
Interstitial Cystitis

My name is Twanna and I have Interstitial Cystitis.

Most of you have probably never heard of it. If you have, you probably have I.C., and wish you hadn't. It is a disease of the bladder where the lining is very thin so your urine is toxic to your bladder. You have the urge to urinate constantly along with great pain. Currently, the medical field has no known cause and therefore no known cure for interstitial cystitis.

I, like everyone else who has been diagnosed with this disease, went through all the approved "torture". I was at the Emergency Room numerous times and was even told by one of the E.R. nurses to pray for death. There was nothing anyone could do for me. I went through cat scans, M.R. I. scans, biopsies, colonoscopies, stomach scopes, and even laparoscopic surgery before I was diagnosed. All this time my pain scale was at 10 always and I grew more depressed every day. The only answer they gave me was bigger and bigger pain pills. At that point and time, I was happy to get them because the pain was always so great.

Then the fun really began and I was sent to an urologist. Don't get me wrong, they were kind to me and did everything they knew how to do. I started having bladder "cocktails". This was a catheter into my bladder 3 times a week for over a year. I was also put on the drug Elmiron. I don't have to describe how the catheters were, if you have ever had one you know. The Elmiron was very expensive even with good insurance. Its side effects were permanent hair loss and damage to your liver (which you had to check every six months). This process helped some but never got my pain below a 6. Everyday life was a struggle. Keeping positive was a struggle.

Then one day on the internet I typed in the search bar *"Hope for Interstitial Cystitis"* and Baker Chiropractic and Wellness came up. I read the whole thing on I.C. and how they have helped many people over the years. Was I skeptical? Yes. Was my family skeptical? Yes. But I wanted to try something other than drugs or the dreaded catheter. What did I have to lose?

So I made an appointment and went in and talked to them. I remember crying through the whole first appointment. They seemed so positive that they would be able to help me even though for three years I was told no one could.

So I started going to them three times a week. Getting adjustments and therapy. Gradually my pain started to decrease. Dr. Baker also had

155

me adjust my diet and put me on anti-inflammatory supplements, both of which have also helped greatly. Now my pain stays between a 1 and 2, which to me is a 90% improvement.

I have my life back! I can work and take vacations. Some days it's like I don't have I.C. at all. If I do have a big flare (which doesn't happen as often as it used to), Dr. Baker is great to get me right in and it usually only takes a small amount of time to get the flare back down. Currently, I still see Dr. Baker twice a week and my goal is to be pain free like his other I.C. patients soon.
I am very thankful to have found Dr. Baker at Baker Chiropractic and Wellness and to have been given a chance for a pain free life without all the drugs and medical procedures.

I also want to thank and commend his staff. They are friendly, sympathetic, kind and knowledgeable and do Dr. Baker's office proud. I also want to say that I listen to the comments between Dr. Baker and his other patients. I hear how much he really cares for them and the gratitude and respect they have for him. All of which is rare in today's world in the medical field. Usually you are just another number.

If you have interstitial cystitis and you have tried everything and nothing is working, or you are tired of taking drugs, give Dr. Baker the chance to help you. You have nothing to lose.

Thanks again to Dr. Baker and his staff. May God bless each and every one of you."

- **Twanna Aldridge**

I was battling Interstitial Cystitis or IC for 3 years before meeting Dr. Paul Baker. When my problem first started, I was on antibiotics a number of times which I believe made my situation worse. I was finally diagnosed with IC and prescribed IC medicine. I tried other procedures too like instillation and dilation every 1 or 2 months for more than a year.

Initially, I could control my symptoms to an extent while on medications but as time passed, nothing helped. I grew very tired of regular visits to the doctor's office and spending lots of money. Finally, I decided to restrict my diet and started regular workouts in order to keep my problem minimized. I had become hopeless about a complete cure for my disease.

One Monday morning, I woke up with a severe IC flare-up and my back was hurting too. I thought I had just pulled a muscle from the work I had done over the weekend and my backache would go away. But I wasn't sure what was aggravating my IC pain. I missed work and school for 4 days and tried everything I could think of at home to alleviate my symptoms. On Thursday morning, I was searching the internet for a doctor in Cincinnati that could treat IC and came across the Baker Chiropractic website.

Although I had my doubts about chiropractic care, I wanted to give it a try. I was already hopeless from failed medical treatments for my IC and on top of it, my back was hurting too. After an X-ray, Dr. Paul told me that I had a subluxation for a very long time and all my symptoms were related. Surprisingly, I actually got some relief after my very first chiropractic adjustment which convinced me to continue adjustments. Dr. Paul also suggested a natural detox solution for everyday use which has become my favorite remedy. Now, I can eat and drink regularly.

Within 2-3 weeks, I was completely symptoms free! It's been 2 months and I don't have any IC troubles anymore. I am still getting adjusted in order to completely correct my spine and keep it healthy. I love the many benefits, some which I didn't even expect. I have a healthier abdomen and my chronic dry eye problem is getting better too.

Thanks to Dr. Paul Baker, I would recommend anyone suffering from Interstitial Cystitis to give Baker Chiropractic a try. I believe they will create wonders for you just like they did for me!

Divya

• • • • •

I have been coming to Baker Chiropractic for a variety of medical problems. I am writing to you and asking you to share with everyone a very embarrassing, debilitating and life changing disease that I was diagnosed with in December, 2009.

You have helped me with so many things that I never even thought to ask you if you and chiropractic adjustments could help me with this disease. In October, 2010, when I truly felt at my lowest as my body was filled with pain, I asked you if you could help me with all the excruciating pain I was having. I was diagnosed with Interstitial Cystitis (IC) after going to two of my doctors and having some uncomfortable testing from both doctors. I remember specifically that I asked you in a "whisper", if you could help me with the IC. I didn't want anyone to hear me asking you because it is very difficult to talk about. I couldn't believe it when you told me you had helped other patients with Interstitial Cystitis and you explained how you do this.

As you know, Interstitial Cystitis can be found in both males and females. In my understanding, the inner lining of the bladder becomes inflamed like it is raw inside. This is a problem with all the different kinds of foods and drinks someone consumes. There is a very strict diet for IC and while on this diet, I felt like I was starving and I was still having painful problems. My doctors told me they had no idea what truly causes it. There is only one medicine available at $365.00 per month, taken three times a day and the minor in-office procedures to help with the pain are expensive as well. The IC is extremely painful and can make you urinate up to 60 times a day and the hardest part is the very painful bladder spasms. This is worse than pregnancy or kidney stones.

Dr. Paul, after two adjustments and your manipulations to the correct area of my spine and the nerves to my bladder...the Interstitial Cystitis and all the pain has stopped!! You still give me adjustments in this area on my regular visits and I can't believe I have my life back again...thanks to you!! I had gotten to the point where I didn't leave my home for weeks at a time and you gave me back my freedom. I have no symptoms at all. The pain and spasms are gone. I can't thank you enough for your help these past four years and especially with the IC. I truly hope your patients that may have this disease can come forward to you and let you heal them as you did for me.

With heartfelt thanks...you are definitely my hero and the best Doctor in the USA!'

- **Judy**

35
Irritable Bowel Syndrome

"At the age of 19, I was diagnosed with Irritable Bowel Syndrome. Being in horrendous pain and discomfort became normal to me.

I am now 26 and throughout the past 7 years, I have seen several doctors and was prescribed 6 different medications.

The only medication that worked was $207 a month with insurance. It made me feel very nauseated and short of breath.

After seeing Dr Paul Baker for 3 chiropractic adjustments, I saw immediate results. I was able to stop taking the medication and canceled the costly appointments with the specialists.

I would also like to add that everyone at the office is incredibly friendly and welcoming!"

- **Lora Stewart**

36
Knee Pain

I became a patient of Dr. Baker on August 5, 2011. I could barely walk and I was considering taking a leave of absence from work. The pain was so bad and I had zero energy.

It all started in 2007 when I hurt my knee. My regular physician sent me to physical therapy for my back. I started taking 2-4 *Aleve* per

165

day. My back felt better but my knee continued to hurt. I began to walk funny because of the knee pain. My whole body got messed up because of my walk.

I was afraid of chiropractic care even though my husband and daughter had been seeing Dr. Baker for over 2 years. I had no choice but to go because by then I had taken more than 2,820 *Aleve* over the span of 4 years. I bought my *Aleve* from Sam's Club in the big 500 count bottles and always carried them with me, but now I don't even think about them. I also took *Benadryl* and *Sudafed* on a regular basis and ever since my first adjustment I no longer have taken either of those. Also, I had only taken 14 *Aleve* in the first 2 months of my chiropractic care.

My x-rays showed that I had no curve in my lower back, my spine was crooked and I had a disk pressing into my spinal cord. I'll be honest – the first 4-6 weeks of my care, I felt worse and wanted to quit. Dr. Baker told me to hang in there and that I wasn't going to get better overnight when it took years to get in this shape. By the 10th week, I had energy and was able to move again. Suddenly the pain was disappearing and I was feeling good. I'm not

100% yet, but I am getting there with regular chiropractic adjustments. My whole life is changing because of it.

I'm 58 years old and not ready to sit in a rocker for the rest of my life. I have 8 grandkids with another on the way and a great grandchild due in March. I want to enjoy life with them. I would definitely recommend to everyone to try chiropractic first before giving up or having surgery. Dr. Baker is fantastic and the girls in the office are so sweet and helpful. They make you feel right at home. And if you hurt at anytime, Olivia and Jess will help with therapy.

My knee feels great now! My husband is a Happy Captain and I am his Happy First Mate. Life is worth living again! Thanks Baker Chiropractic!

- **M. Holbert**

37
Leg Pain

I fell and all my weight was put on my right leg. The pain was so bad that I could not stand on my right leg. I had an MRI, sonogram, x-rays and plenty of pain pills. They didn't help at all.

My friend told me about Dr. Baker and I started going to him. Now, I can walk up and down stairs and no more pain pills!

168

I'm planning on using my new tread mill and playing golf again. Thank you for making me feel good – without pain pills.

- **J. Denny**

38

Medical Doctors Who Are Patients

When I first came to Dr. Paul at Baker Chiropractic, I could hardly walk because my back was in spasm. My residents and medical students had to push me around the hospital in a wheelchair! Using a well-rounded treatment approach including an absolutely painless adjustment, I was 30 percent better in just one visit. By the end of the week, I was walking upright and pain free. All without the need for anti-inflammatory medications, muscle relaxants, or pain pills!

- **B. Masterson, MD**

It is my belief that Chiropractic Medicine is one of the misunderstood, underappreciated, and perhaps, effective treatment modalities available. I attribute my being able to remain off the "disabled list" to Dr. Paul Baker's remarkable clinical skill and knowledge.

- **M. Heintzelman, PH.D.**

Before seeing Dr. Baker I was having pain in my neck and lower back that was radiating into my legs. My activity level and quality of life was quite limited. Now I still feel some occasional discomfort but the pain has subsided and I am now mobile enough to coach my daughter's basketball team and go shopping with my wife. I also really enjoy the family atmosphere in the office. Everyone is so friendly and remembers your name. This helps makes the total experience so pleasant.

- **Dr. S. Thomas**

Just like Drs. Paul and Patrick Baker, I knew at a very young age that I wanted to care for people. I became a medical doctor dedicated to helping people prevent health problems from developing in the first place. As an OB/GYN who has cared for hundreds of expectant mothers and delivered their babies, pregnant women as well as their newborn children can benefit greatly from chiropractic care in the prevention and treatment of many ailments, disorders and diseases. Removing subluxations through chiropractic care enables people of all ages to maximize their health.

M. Pelletier, M.D., C.C.N., F.A.C.O.G.
LaValle Metabolic Institute
Director of Functional Medicine

39
Migraines

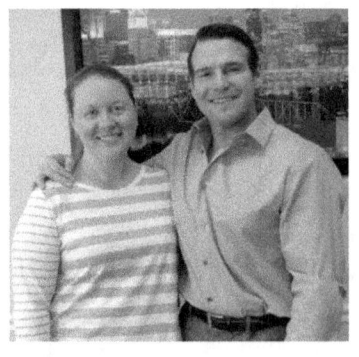

I decided to give chiropractic care a try in August of 2012. When I initially made the appointment to see Dr. Patrick Baker at the Fairfield Clinic, I had no idea that I would still be going a year and a half later or that it would turn out to be such a life-changing decision.

I originally made the appointment because I was having severe neck pain. I could not tilt my head from side to side and I would wake up from sleeping with constant headaches. After the spinal exam and X-ray results were in, I found out that I was suffering from a condition called Forward Head Posture. I have also suffered with migraines since I was thirteen, and Dr. Baker assured me that the chiropractic adjustments would help with those as well. I decided to proceed with Dr. Baker's treatment plan, and it was one of the best choices I have ever made.

After the first couple weeks of adjustments, I noticed a dramatic decrease in the level of neck pain I was experiencing. The constant headaches began to subside, and within a month, I was virtually pain free. And that was just the beginning. I also noticed that I was sleeping better and had more energy. And after just a couple months of care, the migraines became less frequent. I went from having migraines three to four times a month to just three to four times a year in the time I've been a patient.

I wish I would have known years ago how much chiropractic care could help with the migraines alone. I would have started going sooner. And I urge anyone reading this that does get migraines to give it a shot. It will really improve your quality of life, much more so than those triptans we all get when we tell our docs that we get migraines. As if the migraine itself isn't bad enough, we're prescribed pills that only work some of the time and leave us in a sleepy haze for three days afterwards. No thanks. I'll take a massage and an adjustment instead. At least then I know I'm treating the problem and not the symptom – as evidenced by the fact that I no longer get the migraines with any real frequency. And when I do get them, they are much less severe. I no longer take triptans to treat them.

Or any prescription medicine, for that matter. Since I had been feeling so much better, I asked Dr. Baker to help me with stepping down off the antidepressant I had been prescribed three years ago because I had no lingering symptoms of depression and I felt like the meds were keeping me in a constant fog. He referred me to Dr. Theodore Cole at the Cole Center for Healing, and with their help, I was able to successfully step down of the medicine two months ago without any side effects. Except a little weight loss.

Which brings me to the bonus: since attending the Baker Chiropractic Total Food Makeover seminar in February of 2013 and slowly implementing the nutrition and fitness guidelines that were provided, I have lost 40 pounds. And I'm still losing!

That's what I have enjoyed so much about this whole experience. It has been nothing but positive, and the doctors and staff are truly invested in helping you achieve your health goals. They take the time to educate you and provide you with the tools that you need to succeed. I am grateful to all of them for their help and support. I don't even want to think about what my quality of life would be like right now had I not decided to seek chiropractic care. So if you're thinking about giving it a try, just go for it. It will be one of the best decisions you ever make.

Amanda Grow

My teenage son awoke one morning with blurred vision and sensitivity to light. I attributed it to lack of sleep or too much "screen time", and insisted that he go to school. I also knew that we had a scheduled visit with an ophthalmologist in a few days. It had been nearly two years since his eyes had been checked and he was overdue for new lenses.

Not long after arriving at school, he reported to the nurse with a debilitating headache. I brought him home where he spent the rest of the day on the living room sofa in the dark. I took him to the pediatrician that evening. The pediatrician looked into his eyes with a scope and had him read an eye chart. We were sent directly to the emergency room of a Children's Hospital. After four hours and a phone call to a neurologist, the staff pediatrician looked into my son's eyes with a scope and had him read an eye chart. The consensus was that he had a migraine headache.

We pretty much suspected that, but I was concerned about the sudden onset of blurred vision, as it might indicate something was immediately going wrong in his brain, like a concussion, aneurysm tumor ... parents think like that, right?

We were relieved to finally be dismissed from the ER, with orders for my son to take a pain reliever and get a good night's sleep. If the headaches persisted, we should consult a neurologist who could prescribe a drug for migraine headaches.

The next morning, my son awoke with blurred vision, extreme sensitivity to light, and pain in the back of his head. The next day was another day on the sofa, taking pain relievers and no school.

Day three went pretty much the same way, except we made a visit to our chiropractor, Dr. Paul Baker. Dr. Paul told us that his C2 vertebrae was subluxated. After one adjustment, the relief was immediate. After two chiropractic treatments, neck traction with a Dakota cushion at home, good nutrition, sleep and back to drinking the recommended daily amount of water, my son's migraine headaches have not returned.

We continue our regular visits to Dr. Paul. He and the staff treat us like family. The care is genuine and the results are real. My son has new glasses, too. He likes to research topics on the internet. He learned that approximately 20% of teenagers are affected by migraine headaches. Drugs prescribed for migraines can have serious effects on the liver and heart. The ocular nerve that affects vision is located by the C2 vertebrae.

Poor posture from staring at a computer screen for long periods can cause subluxations in your spine. We are so grateful to have Dr. Baker straighten things out for us.

Drug free, real cures. That's what Baker Family Chiropractic is all about.

- **Kimberly Flick and son Jerry**

• • • • •

When I was seventeen years old I fractured my neck and two bones in my back. I was very lucky that I wasn't hurt worse than I was. I went through six months of being in a neck cast, 8 hours of surgery, and then six additional months of physical therapy. Pain was a daily issue for me. My muscles were so tight that I would constantly have migraines. I couldn't focus. There would be days that I would just shut the whole world out, and go to a dark quiet place just to find some sort of relief, but still there was none.

One day, my Mom told me to go to Dr. Baker since he has helped everyone in my family. I thought ok, I'll give it a try. Why not? That was the best decision I could have ever made. Within one week I could tell a difference. Within a month I was headache free.

Something that I never thought would happen. I could actually enjoy life again. I can't even put a price on that. Words cannot describe how grateful I am to Dr. Baker and his staff. They gave me my life back.

-   **Brittany Brewer (Weaver)**

40
Multiple Sclerosis (MS)

Dear Dr. Baker and Staff - We have been regular patients at your Fairfield office for over ten years now and are very happy with our experiences there. You and your staff are always friendly and helpful in addition to efficient in administering effective treatments.

Cindy's experiences:

I was diagnosed with multiple sclerosis (MS) in the early 1990s and my mobility gradually decreased for several years. Physical therapy routines and medications helped to suspend my physical decline at a point where I have limited mobility (use wheelchair, walker, hand-holds, etc.). After finding physical therapy alone was not enough to maintain my mobility, I decided to try chiropractic therapy.

My neurologist is supportive of chiropractic treatment to manage the effects of MS, and I believe regular chiropractic treatments are allowing me to maintain my limited mobility by keeping the parts of my body I over-use or under-use in a flexible state rather than allowing them to atrophy.

I have been treated regularly by Dr. Baker for about 15 years now, and this has helped me maintain my mobility at a stable level. These regular treatments also help to avoid and provide relief from occasional bouts of sciatic nerve pain (probably indirectly associated with the MS). I believe it likely I would be confined to a wheelchair without these regular chiropractic treatments.

I have also observed a decrease in mobility with time when I am unable to receive my regular chiropractic treatments. I believe chiropractic treatments are making a significant difference in my quality of life with MS.

Tony's experiences:

I have always been fairly active. I used to play softball regularly, I bowl regularly, I coached outdoor sports for my sons, I golf occasionally and go on occasional fishing marathons, in addition to the normal yard work etc. associated with maintaining a home.

Previous to regular chiropractic treatment, I would periodically (1-2 times/year) experience painful and debilitating pinched nerve problems in my upper back/shoulder area. These were treated with muscle relaxing drugs before I began visiting Dr. Baker.

I have not experienced a single pinched nerve incident during the approximately 15 years I have been treated by Dr. Baker. This is amazing to me, and I am definitely happy with these results!

Thanks – and keep up the good work!

- **Tony and Cindy Dowrey**

41

Neck and Shoulder Pain

I couldn't move my neck and was overweight by more than 30 pounds. I didn't feel very good about myself as a person.

Now, I feel 100% better. I also believe chiropractic care is so much better than traditional medicine. If doctors in traditional medical practices approached their careers,

186

their practices and most importantly their patients with the same attitude and work ethic as Dr. Baker, my attitude might be different.

Thank you Dr. Baker for being there for me and providing a much needed change in my life.

- **D. Krause**

I came to see Dr. Baker because I was having trouble with my neck. I sit all day at a computer and my fingers in my right hand were going numb. I knew from past chiropractic care from another doctor the problem I was experiencing was from my neck. After several adjustments I was feeling so much better. While talking to Dr. Baker he told me that he could help me with my headaches and shoulder pain. This was something I thought I would have to live with the rest of my life.

My headaches were so frequent my primary care Doctor was having me log them so we could try to figure out what was triggering them. After several adjustments I am happy to say I am not suffering from them anymore.

My shoulders were so rounded forward I did not realize how bad they were. Now with Dr. Bakers help they are almost back to normal and my posture is so much better.

I like the way Dr. Baker takes into account the whole body. I came in for one problem and he has helped me so much more. I can't thank Dr. Baker and his staff enough for helping me feel better and have a better quality of life.

- **J. Johnson**

42

Neurocardiogenic Syncope

 I first came to Doc because of continual back pain. At my consultation I mentioned that I have a condition the doctors have labeled neurocardiogenic syncope, which causes me to faint frequently. I had never met anyone who had experience with this until Doc informed me that he has handled patients with this: he was sure he could help. I can't say that I believed him right away, but that has changed!

One Sunday I had two episodes and continued to suffer from vertigo and pain into Monday. I went to Doc's that afternoon and in just one adjustment my dizziness subsided! He sent me for a massage, where his staff eased a lot of the pain and the headache. I was amazed and so thankful!

- **S. Dickman**

43

Osteoporosis

I am 81 years old and had a lot of constant pain. The tests and x-rays showed osteoporosis, scoliosis and osteoarthritis. My medical doctor told me all this caused high blood pressure and prescribed a blood pressure pill.

I began to get completely bent over and had to walk sideways. I would visit the YMCA two or three times per week and exercise in the pool which would help loosen me up.

My daughter made an appointment for me at Baker Chiropractic. My first visit showed my x-ray was a "mess". I am now showing improvements and have faith in this health care practice. I can drive and I can live on my own. Without these caring and dedicated people, I would be in a nursing home. God Bless them!

-   **A. Gillespie**

44
Pinched Nerve

Rich Pohana suffered from a severe pinched nerve in his back causing back pain, psoas pain and calf pain. After undergoing corrective chiropractic care, he was able to go on and complete the "Death Valley" bike ride and hike.

Rich rode his bike 148 miles, a ride up 13,403 ft of vertical elevation and hiked on foot 11 miles which took him up another 6,140 feet of vertical elevation. Rich stood on top of the

mountain and proudly held his Baker
Chiropractic Shirt high!

LOW (ELV. -282 FT.) TO HIGH (ELV. 14,505 FT.)
Badwater to Mt. Whitney Portal By Bicycle
•148 miles 13,403 ft. of vertical elevation

Mt. Whitney Portal to Summit On Foot
•11 miles 6,140 ft. of vertical elevation

Temperature Differential of 100+ degrees F (including wind chill factor)

*Thanks
Dr. Paul*

45

Professional Athletes Who are Patients

I played with a left hamstring injury since playing college football at Washington University. I went to doctors all over the country to find out what was wrong, and none of the doctors could figure out the problem in my hamstring. I went to Drs. Baker and they found a huge knot in my hamstring and they were able to release it and fix my hamstring problem that I have had since college. I now get adjusted before and after every game. I have been injury free for the past 3 years and have been to the last three Pro Bowls.

- **Corey Dillon, NFL Pro Bowl Running Back**

Playing in the NFL is very physically demanding on my lower back. Over the last two years of getting adjusted by the Bakers, my lower back has felt 100% better. My lower back is more flexible and strong. I've been injury free since I have been getting adjusted.

- **Brian Simmons, Cincinnati Bengals Linebacker**

I have never felt better since getting my back adjusted and getting my hamstrings released before and after each game. Since I have been under regular Chiropractic care with Drs. Baker I have been more resilient to injuries and much more flexible. Getting adjusted before and after each game has made a huge difference in my performance

- **Adrian Ross, NFL Linebacker**

I have been a professional bodybuilder for over ten years and I have literally injured almost every joint and muscle in my body. I have been getting adjusted and massaged at Baker Family Chiropractic regularly for the past two years and I can't tell you what a difference it has made in my life. My neck, shoulders and back feel so much better after getting adjusted. I am able to train with as much intensity now as I did when I was 25 years old. Thanks for all your help Doctors.

- **Franco Santoriello, IFBB Professional Body Builder**

46

Restless Leg Syndrome (RLS)

I started coming to Baker Chiropractic in October of 2013.

I had trouble with my hands - numbness (but not going totally numb) and tingling about three years ago. My family doctor said it was probably Carpel Tunnel since I was not a diabetic. I just took it for that because it only happened at night and not all the time. Then last year in January of 2013 my feet and legs started with the same tingling, numbness, burning...mostly at night.

I started reading up on the causes of Neuropathy. Oh my gosh, I thought I was going to have something really bad wrong with me. I made another appointment with my family doctor and he told me to go see a neurologist, which I did.

They did testing on me finding out that I did not have Carpel Tunnel or nerve damage in my hands, legs or feet. So he said that I might have Restless Leg Syndrome (RLS) and gave me a prescription for a medication that helps people with RLS. He said he didn't know what was wrong with my hands and that I could get RLS in my hands. REALLY?! So I started on the medication. I also started doing all kinds of research on what causes Restless Leg Syndrome and neuropathy along with all the different things I could do to help it get better.

I TRIED EVERYTHING. I started taking more vitamins. Doctor also said I might have a vitamin B-6 or B-12 deficiency, so I started taking those along with my fish oil and my cholesterol medication (low dose). After about three to four months there was no difference in the way I was feeling.

I now had the tingling, numbness and burning all through the day. I was desperate and thought I was going to have to live like this for the rest of my life. So back to the research. One of my daughter-in laws suggested I should try a chiropractor. I thought what the heck. I've tried everything else, but like others was skeptical about a chiropractor.

I started looking for chiropractors close to where I worked so I could go during the day. I was looking at different websites and found Baker Chiropractic and Wellness. I got on their website, got their number and called. I talked to Danielle and she said "Oh yes we can help" and made me an appointment.

Still skeptical, I went to my first appointment. They did x-rays of my back and neck. Then, I had a consultation with Dr. Baker. Boy was I a mess.....worse than what I could have ever imagined.

He said, "Harvy I can help you, it took you a long time to get this way and it will take awhile to get things back in place". I had pinched nerves in my upper back that caused tingling in my hands. My back was really bad and he said that was the problem with my feet and hands. It all had to do with my nerves!

My husband and I went to the presentation that he gives all new patients and he explained how everything is connected to your spinal cord and nerves and what everything does. WOW, what an eye opener!

Well, I started my first appointment (adjustment) the next week. Dr. Baker had wanted me to come three times a week to start, but I could only come two days a week. By my third adjustment, the tingling and numbness in my hands was almost gone. Now they hardly bother me. AWESOME!

Everyone at Baker Chiropractic is so nice and helpful, they are wonderful.

Both Dr. Patrick and Dr. Paul are always asking how you are doing and REALLY care about you and what you are feeling. You can really tell they care and will try to do everything to make things better. They listen and take the time to answer your questions or concerns and offer suggestions on things to do. They encourage you and explain why this or that might be happening.

My legs and feet are much better than before. There are some days (several days) when they don't bother me at all. I still have my days with the left side of my leg and feet, BUT NOTHING LIKE BEFORE. .AWESOME!

THEY DEFINITELY HAVE A GIFT FROM GOD... Healing in their hands.

THANK YOU SO MUCH Dr. Patrick, Dr. Paul and everyone at Baker Chiropractic and Wellness for helping me feel better again.

- **Harvy Thomas**

47
Sciatica Pain

"I walked into Baker Chiropractic with a sciatic pain attack from a compressed disc. I thought I would never recover. I have never experienced pain like this. The pain was worse than labor pains!

Dr. Paul Baker told me with treatment I would get better. I had a friend that had an attack the same time as I and to date is still in pain and considering surgery.

So back to my story, Dr. Paul gave me my treatment four times a week which included adjustments and massage therapy.

I can tell you that I was unable to sit, stand, walk or lay on my side when I first came to Dr. Paul. Five weeks later, I was doing all of these things.

My nerves calmed down, my inflammation was reduced and all without pain or muscle relaxers. My treatment plan was the key.

I would recommend Dr. Paul, Baker Chiropractic and the entire staff to anyone. Without this group of caring people, I would probably have had an unnecessary surgery at a high expense.

Thank God for Baker Chiropractic!"

- **Phyllis Holliman**

Last year, nearing the age of 70 I had three choices: 1. Have a back operation, 2. Use a cane and wheelchair or 3. Live my life on pain pills. Being an active grandmother of four this wasn't on my agenda. Doctors told me there were discs pinching my nerves that were causing sciatica pain to travel down my left leg into my foot.

Excruciating migraine headaches also caused more pain creating the need for pain pills. I decided to try one more thing desperately hoping it would work. After limping into the office of Baker Chiropractic and filling out a medical form, one question being, on a scale of 1-10, ten being severe, what is your level of pain? Mine was 10 and 1/2. After giving me an x-ray and discussing my problems Dr. Paul Baker told me that he could eliminate my pain and I would have no need for pain pills.

Within the first few visits there was definite relief. The exercises, therapy and adjustments caused the migraines to go away first. My leg was a different story though. With each visit Dr. Paul assured me that the pain didn't occur overnight and that he would correct my problem. I have come to find out that as one matures it takes a little longer to heal. Due to Dr. Paul's continued expertise in releasing muscle tightness, knowledge of the body and continuing adjustments my pain level has decreased 95%, which he has told me will be down to 0 very shortly.

Now I can walk 3 miles every day, shop at the mall for 4 hours, dance with my granddaughters (taught them how to jitterbug) and take vacations requiring sitting for long periods of time, without the need of pain pills. Dr. Paul and his staff are very friendly and efficient. I sing their praises to all my friends and truly thank the day I walked into the office of Baker Chiropractic.

-   **G. McGurrin**

48

Scoliosis

 My name is Kristin Betsch and even though I am only eighteen years old, I have been living with chronic back pain most of my life. I had gone to doctor after doctor, and that eventually led to surgeons. I was diagnosed with scoliosis when I was about ten years old and have been monitored ever since. I was told

208

scoliosis does not cause back pain, but there was no other explanation. The last straw was when they referred me to pain management, this was their final solution. But first, I put my foot down. I stood up for myself and said there was no way I would take pain medication the rest of my life. That's when I found Baker Chiropractic. This practice and all of their staff was truly God-send. It was slow going at first, but I never gave up hope. I don't know where I would be or how I would feel today if I hadn't found Doctor Baker. Now, I don't just get my back adjusted, but anything else you can think of, I get adjusted also. I finally physically feel my age! So THANK YOU to all the staff at Baker Chiropractic, you saved my life!

Hi, my name is Lauren. In 2002, I was

diagnosed with scoliosis and a 90 degree spinal curve. It was so bad that traditional medical care was not helping.

In 2011, I went on-line and found Dr. Paul Baker at Baker

Chiropractic and Wellness.
Baker Chiropractic's mission is to empower families to take charge of their own health without using drugs, surgeries or other invasive procedures.
I called for an appointment the next day which consisted of a consultation and an exam.

Dr. Paul Baker and his staff were so welcoming and knowledgeable that I knew this was the right place for me.

I have been going to Dr. Paul for 3 years and counting. It's been an amazing experience!
He has helped me with so many things that I had no idea chiropractic care could help with.

In February of this year (2014), I had new x-rays taken and the results were shocking. The curve from my scoliosis was reduced to 50 degrees!

- **Lauren Mantoufe**

My name is Karen Tribby and I came to Baker Chiropractic because I was having trouble with my back and trouble walking. I have been diagnosed with osteopina; complications from having scoliosis and TMJ in my left upper jawbone.

I went to see Dr. Patrick Baker because I noticed he helped my co-worker, Craig Boykin with his back and walking. Craig has cerebral palsy and he has trouble with his arm being paralyzed and joints that just do not move as they should. I thought if he could help Craig, then maybe I had a chance for help.

I have been to three medical doctors in the past for other medical problems and none helped. It is very frustrating for me because when you have a serious medical problem and you hear the words, "no help", it is hard to keep your faith in doctors and people in general. To add to my problems, I have a ventro-jugular shunt that is in my skull and I was not sure if Dr. Baker had ever heard of or worked with this type of medical procedure. I was born with hydrocephalus and this is why I have the shunt.

When I first met Dr. Patrick Baker and his staff, I noticed that they are very positive people and are committed to helping their patients live normal and healthy lives.
I began my road to a healthier life with Baker Chiropractic in October, 2011. It has been one year now and I have had amazing results with movement returned to my back, legs, neck and shoulders. I did not realize that these areas were being affected by my back. I will continue my road to a healthier life with Baker Chiropractic for years to come. I want to live my elderly years being healthy and very active. Thank you very much to Dr. Patrick Baker and his staff, may you continue to keep doing what you do and help people live a much healthier lifestyle!

- **Karen Tribby**

49
Shoulder Injury

"When I first met Dr. Patrick Baker it was at AutoZone. I was recently coming off losing a football scholarship due to a shoulder injury. I was pretty down about everything. I had gone through a year of rehab and I still couldn't do push-ups or bench press or anything related to my shoulders.

When I was talking to Doc, I explained that to him. He started telling me there was a possibility that I had pinched nerves and it wasn't allowing everything to heal properly. I was very skeptical but I thought to myself what could it hurt. We set up an appointment and that was the beginning of my healing.

After my first visit, I felt on top of the world. I had more energy. I went home and did my first push up in a year and half. On my following visit, I told Dr. Baker about that. He told me I'm on the road to being maximized. After about a month of regular chiropractic care, I could do around 25 pushups. I was back to bench pressing 135 lbs.

I'm now about 6 months into Dr. Baker's care and I have received another football scholarship. I have a shot at making it to the pros. I firmly believe that if God would have never sent Dr. Baker and the family at Baker Chiropractic, I wouldn't be able to play football again.

So the skepticism for me and chiropractic care has completely been lifted. I would recommend anyone with an injury to give it a go. It's well worth it!"

- **Robert Mincey #84**

50
Spinal Bifida

I am 43 years old. I was born with Spinal Bifida. I have had 42 surgeries. I have been going to the Baker Brothers for 10 years or more. I go at least 2 or 3 times a week and it is the only thing that is keeping me out of a wheel chair. Trust me when it comes to the effectiveness of chiropractic care.

216

Having so much pain and joints hurt, there are times the pain goes away for a little while and it is a great day for me. I can get something done at home for a little while or go to the store for shopping and bring the groceries in and it takes a day for me to do this. Then there are days I hurt all over and cannot get anything done.

But I know I have an appointment the next day and just getting adjusted gives me a day back and sometimes the next day I feel like a new person for a while like I can do anything because I know I will have another appointment waiting for me and I can make it through another day.

Thanks to the Baker Brothers! I am still wheel chair free at 43 and still going!

-   **P. Tuttle**

51
Tachycardia

"I began being treated at Baker Chiropractic and Wellness in the early part of July. My initial complaint was about a small curve that I noticed forming in my upper back.
Once I was in the office I was given a diagram of the spine. In this diagram it showed how the

spine is connected to everything in the body. I already knew this, but I never really knew about it in depth. Once given the diagram and speaking with Dr. Paul Baker, I was educated on how the curve in my spine was affecting my body.

Oddly enough I had been having some small troubles with my heart a few months prior to coming to Dr. Baker. I had not mentioned this to anyone in the office. Once Dr. Baker finished explaining to me what his findings were I asked him if the heart problems I had been experiencing could be coming from the curve in my back. His response to me was "absolutely."

He explained that the spine is attached to everything in the body, and what I probably had going on was a pinched nerve that lead straight to my heart. This made total sense to me because I had already undergone a series of tests that revealed nothing. I was put on medications that I felt I really shouldn't be taking being that the doctor really didn't know what was causing my ailment.

Dr. Baker began my exercises and adjustments immediately. After about 5 visits I have already noticed a change. My heart ailment is not as pronounced anymore. I am able to sleep. I am not as irritable as I had been over the past few months. Going to the chiropractor for this short time has given me faster results than going to the medical doctor for all of those months. I feel like the medication I was given was to treat my symptoms but Dr. Baker is treating and correcting the problem.

I am so glad I made the decision to go to the chiropractor when I did. Dr. Baker is so honest and warm. Once you encounter him you know that he is genuine and that he is determined to help you to the best of his ability. His staff is the same way. By my second visit they all knew me by name. In a place where they see hundreds of patients a day this was impressive. They have always greeted me by name and with a smile. If I have any questions or concerns I have no problems being helped.

I LOVE Dr. Baker and his staff. They have truly changed my life."

- **Elease North**

52
Temporomandibular Joint Disorder TMJ

I don't remember when it started. But it's safe to say that I have had TMJ for a long time... for most of my life.

I had it long before I had a name for it. It

221

was simply that clicky-jaw-thing. And by clicky-jaw-thing, I mean that thing when you yawn or chew or laugh really hard and your jaw pops... loudly. And someone near you says, "What was that?!" And then you say, "Oh... that was my jaw." Not so much topic of conversation and pretty humiliating.

The clicky-jaw-thing stuck around through all of high school and into college before I knew that there was actually a technical term for it. I finally asked the dentist about it and he said that the clicking was caused by a Temporomandibular Joint disorder, or TMJ. Basically, he said that my jaw was out of line. He suggested a night mouth guard because TMJ can sometimes be caused by nighttime teeth grinding and I was a confirmed teeth grinder.

Over the years, I used a mouth guard from the dentist, bought several from different drug stores, and had another made by a different dentist. They made me talk funny and drool more, but none of them magically aligned my jaw.

At this point, over ten years ago, my dentist was out of options that didn't require surgery.

I had no intention of getting jaw surgery and at some point in the last decade I had simply resigned myself to the fact that I would be stuck with TMJ for the rest of my life. Unfortunately, this acceptance included frequent headaches, many doses of ibuprofen, and the all too familiar clicky-jaw-thing.

About six months ago we started seeing Dr. Paul. My husband stumbled upon his name (and by stumbled, I mean divine intervention) and went in for an issue he was having with his back and within a few weeks, our daughters and I were also patients. After the back x-rays were taken, the consultation, and the adjustments, I was feeling great, but it didn't even dawn on me to bring up the TMJ. He's a chiropractor, not a dentist... right?

But then I saw him working on a young woman's jaw. And then I heard another young woman tell him how much better her TMJ has been. I nearly cried. I asked Dr. Paul if he worked on TMJ... of course he does! It's been about three months since he started working on my jaw— just a few minutes after each adjustment— and it has already made a remarkable difference!

I used to get headaches every day. Every day. Many of them would start in my jaw and work their way up to my temples. Frequently I would wake up with a searing headache that was lodged primarily in my jaw.

That is a rare occurrence these days. I rarely have headaches and when I do they are slight not severe. My jaw still clicks, but it doesn't send the jolt of pain that it used to. And I have a larger range of motion... which is to say, I can open my mouth wider without the clicking and the hurting.

The pain lifted steadily. It was a release and an overwhelming relief. As I look back, it is baffling that I had accepted that level of discomfort. But when it started to recede and then go away completely, it was like an entirely new life. Having lived with constant pain and to then watch it disappear, I began to realize just how stressful and all-consuming living with that agony had been. The lightness, relief, and joy that come from its lifting are life changing.

Finding Baker Chiropractic, Dr. Paul, and the entire staff has changed the lives of our entire family. We are healthier, happier, and we feel better than ever! Occasionally I imagine how much Advil it would have taken to get through my life with TMJ, or I think about having to endure a painful jaw surgery or wear some contraption on my face every night while I sleep... and each time I send up a silent prayer for Dr. Paul and the path that led us to him.

53

Tremors and Seizures

My son has experienced tremors since birth. They were mild and infrequent until last year. His pediatrician was never able to precisely diagnose his conditions. We went through numerous tests without any conclusions. Before we began treatment at Baker Chiropractic, he had increased his tremor spells to 4-10 times almost daily.

Since we began treatment at Baker Chiropractic, he has had only 2 or 3 tremors and no tremors whatsoever since January.

We were very skeptical at first but now we wish we would have found Dr. Paul and Dr. Patrick earlier.

- **T. Lind**

. . . . .

I was having seizures due to a brain tumor and suffering from severe headaches. I was feeling terrible and was beginning to think that I would have to live life around this pain and stop doing the things I love to do because the pain was so intense. At times, it was unbearable.

After coming to Baker Chiropractic, I began to feel better. The many benefits I have experienced personally from chiropractic care are minimal number of seizures. When I do have them, they don't last as long as before. My headaches are almost entirely diminished and my back pain is much better.

In all honesty, I would have to say I feel better health wise than I have felt in years.

- **O. Murrell**

54
Torticollis

 When Brooke was three months old she was diagnosed with torticollis. Torticollis is the tightening of the muscles on one side of the neck causing the baby to look in only one direction. She was referred to start physical therapy right away.

During our first visit with the PT, we were told torticollis could also cause a flattening of the skull on one side or the back of the head, known as Plagiocephaly. This looked like the direction we were heading, which would result in Brooke wearing a helmet for six months; 23 hours a day.

When we started physical therapy they said it would take at least eight months to see any real improvement. Mind you, we were dealing with a very uncomfortable, fussy baby which called for many sleepless nights. More importantly, how would this condition affect her development; her motor skills.

Eight months seemed like an eternity. I was so discouraged and felt really helpless. One day I was talking to our home health care nurse about Brooke's condition and how I was feeling. She told me her neighbor's son also had torticollis and was treated by Baker Chiropractic. She said he was much more comfortable and sleeping a lot better and recommended I give them a call.
I was a little skeptical. I had heard so many different opinions of chiropractic care, but at

this point was willing to try anything. I can honestly say this is the best thing I could have done for her. After only 10 visits, there is a dramatic improvement in Brooke's condition. She is like a totally different baby. To look at her now you would never know there was ever anything wrong with her. She holds her head straight, looks in either direction, (sleeps thru the night!!!) and is a much much happier baby. Needless to say, I am a much happier mommy!!

I recently took Brooke back to the PT and they themselves were quite impressed with the progress. Turns out, she won't need that helmet after all. To go from facing eight long months of therapy, to results after 10 adjustments is such a relief and truly amazing. I was so afraid we would miss out on the joy of our baby's first year.

I cannot say enough how grateful we are to Dr. Baker and his staff. Everyone there has been so great to work with. They are always so friendly and genuinely happy to see us. As a mother of four little ones walking into a doctor's office, that's not usually the response I get.
Thank you so much for your dedication in helping Brooke. You have given us back those

eight months and lifted a great weight off of our family - I just can't thank you enough for that!!

-   **S. Garrison**

• • • • •

 After much speculation and debate, I decided to succumb to the circumstances and pay Dr. Baker a visit. My newborn daughter, Kendall, had severe feeding issues in that she would spit up most of what she ate at every feeding. In the hospital she would gag and gasp for air it was so severe. I was told that she was having these issues because she was born in less than 40 minutes and it was too quick for fluids to leave her system naturally through the birthing process, and that it would soon cease. After nearly one month of this happening I took her to the pediatrician who diagnosed her with severe acid reflux and prescribed Zantac.

Administering this medicine (for the short time in which I did) was the cruelest thing I have done to any of my children. Although it did seem as if it helped slightly with her gagging and the reflux, the medicine itself was so potent that it would burn my eyes upon smelling it. When I (attempted) to give it to her she would gag, hold her breath and spit it right back at me, and her eyes would water also. After only a few doses, I didn't feel like the side effects of the medicine were worth the benefits, and that there had to be a better alternative. It was then that I was recommended to see Doc.

The more I thought about Kendall's upcoming chiropractic experience, I began to think of other concerns I had. She was always holding her head to one side, and never seemed to develop neck muscles and head control as my other children had at her age. I wasn't quite sure if this was a cause for worry, but it was definitely something that I wanted to address. Our initial meeting with Doc was comforting, informative, and assuring. He addressed all of my questions, and assured me that this was my first step toward living a happier, healthier life for Kendall, I, and the rest of my family.

I was informed that Kendall had a case of Torticollis, and that with adjustments I would see great improvement. So I entrusted Dr. Baker, a father of small children himself, with one of my precious gifts from God and put her health and her future in his hands. For her first adjustment my initial nervousness quickly subsided as I witnessed something amazing. He held her softly between his hands and did his work, and as he did so, she smiled at him and cooed softly putting me to ease. She thoroughly enjoyed what she was experiencing and there seemed to be a weight lifted off my shoulders. Later that night Kendall was in great spirits, and seemed to be less fussy that usual. She was also holding her head up slightly better than usual. I initially played this off as coincidence until our return visits with Doc.

The next time we went, I decided to get adjusted – after all, I had chronic back problems from a wreck and my 50lb+ weight gain from all of my pregnancies had not helped! I walked out of his office feeling like a new person. Instead of walking around and living with a constant ache, I felt something that could not be expressed in words – I literally felt nothing. Kendall and I visited Doc on a regular basis and after just a few visits Kendall's acid reflux had seen a tremendous improvement, and she was holding her head upright as if there had never been a problem. But, most importantly for the both of us, she began sleeping for more than three hours in a row!

My other children have also begun reaping the benefits of chiropractic. My youngest son Kayden, who is two, saw Doc for the first time after an accident in which he received several staples in his head. Doc initially adjusted his neck, but after gaining Kayden's comfort and confidence, he adjusted his back as well. On several occasions Kayden has asked for "Doc to fix neck", and we went to see him!! He even knows the routine and sits patiently in his chair, hands in his lap, for his turn, and then runs to the table and positions himself accordingly for his back adjustments. My five-year-old daughter and son both have been adjusted and they too, have asked on several occasions to see Doc when they were not feeling well. My husband is a landscaper and does snow removal and is constantly on his feet, and constantly saying how badly his back feels. After just one visit he felt tremendously better, and will be returning especially with the grueling winter months ahead of him!

There is no stereotypical chiropractic patient. We come from different backgrounds with different prior experiences, different symptoms, and different goals for relief. Everyone can truly benefit from chiropractic, as I have learned over the past few months, especially with my own family. We all have different symptoms and concerns ranging from acid reflux, constipation, head and neck trauma, ADHD, ear infections, and more! And yet, we all unite under one common ground, that being relief we seek from visiting with Dr. Baker. I have suggested to several family members and friends the benefits they too could achieve. I would never force or insist chiropractic care upon anyone. I would however, ask that anyone and everyone simply try it one time, and let it speak for itself. They too, would be a life-long patient of Baker Chiropractic!

- **The Cortright Family**

55
Vertigo

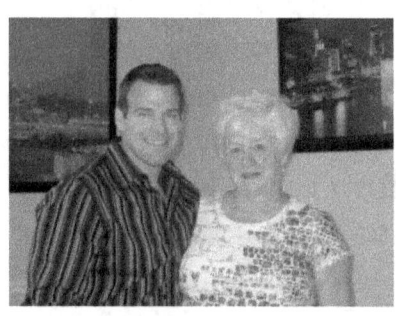

I have been coming to Dr. Patrick Baker since March. Prior to becoming a patient, I experienced constant and severe pain as well as dizziness. However, those symptoms are no longer an issue!

I used to take muscle relaxers and pain medicine, but since I've been coming to Dr. Baker's office I no longer need them. The constant pain would sometimes keep me awake at night. Now I am sleeping better and without pain. At home, I would leave certain chores go undone because I was unable to do them without having severe pain. That has been changed around since becoming a patient. Now I feel like I am actually accomplishing things at home.

There were many days at work where I would actually pray to get through my shift because the pain was so intense. However, I am no longer having that problem because most of the pain has subsided.

Another issue I had prior to becoming a patient was vertigo. Every time I would turn my head, I felt very dizzy. It became a regular occurrence but after getting adjusted, the dizziness stopped.

The added bonus of being Dr. Baker's patient is that he and his staff are all wonderful! I feel like I have gained a bunch of new friends!

- **S. Thomas**

56
Weight Loss & Medication Reduction

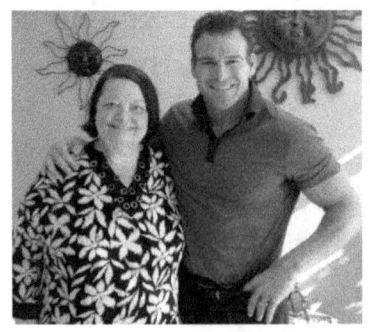

At the end of 2011, Betty Higgins embarked on a unique journey with Baker Chiropractic and Wellness **to** lose weight and gain her health.

At 55 years of age, Betty had struggled with her weight for decades. That battle was taking a toll on her overall physical and mental health. She suffered from a long list of health conditions from fibromyalgia to depression to high cholesterol and was taking thirteen (13) different prescription medications to treat the symptoms of her various ailments. The list included such common prescription medications as:

• Lyrica
• Celebrex
• Lipitor
• Allegra
• Atenolol

Betty had tried all types of diets in the past including the ones that are highly advertised on television by celebrity spokespeople. However, those diets failed her and left her frustrated. She needed something different. She found the difference when she stopped into the Red Bank Clinic of Baker Chiropractic one day and talked to Dr. Paul Baker.

"I felt a strong leading from the Lord just to stop in (the clinic) without an appointment", stated Betty. "They took me right into this bustling office, just liked I belonged there. The rest is history", she added.

Betty had a strong desire to change her health and her life, but she had not found the right program with the right support. Unlike the highly publicized diet plans, Dr. Paul's and Dr. Patrick's LifeCall Weight Loss and Health Gain program is not focused solely on weight loss. In fact, loss of weight is simply a derivative of their unique program.

A LifeCall is about making changes to your lifestyle in order to gain health and lose the elements in your life that are preventing you from having good health.

When Betty started her LifeCall program in 2011, this is what she said about why she was doing it:

"I would like to be able to take better care of my grandchildren. I haven't mentioned it to my daughter, but the reason I won't take both grandchildren outside to play together my myself is that I'm afraid a four year old and a two year old will outrun me and I couldn't keep them safe. I'm ashamed to say that, but it's true. I came to Cincinnati from a failed marriage which in part was caused by my obesity. I would like to regain my health and my life."

In November 2011, Betty sat down with Dr. Paul Baker and Dr. Patrick Baker to discuss her LifeCall program. They provided her with detailed plan to escape her unhealthy habits and develop a new and healthier way of life.

The doctors showed Betty how to eat, taught her the importance of proper nutrition, provided her with guidance on exercise and set a schedule of regular chiropractic care with Dr. Paul.

Betty's first steps in her LifeCall program began by throwing out all the processed foods in her refrigerator and pantry that were providing her with little or no nutrition. Then, she went on a special shopping tour at a local supermarket where she was showed what food to buy and what to look for on the labels. The doctors also gave her a detailed exercise plan to follow along with regular chiropractic care.

For the last twelve months, Betty has been following the LifeCall program, attending routine chiropractic care with Dr. Paul and enjoying the support and motivation of the Baker Chiropractic and Wellness staff. Her investment in herself is paying huge dividends. Here's what Betty has accomplished:

• **Lost 70 lbs. of weight.**
• **Reduced dependency on prescription medications from 13 to 3.**
• **Self esteem restored.**
• **Confidence increased.**
• **Positive outlook on the future.**

"If someone would have told me I would be 70lbs. lighter in one year, I would not have believed them", said an overjoyed Betty Higgins. "I had tried to lose weight and keep it off for 30 years and had lost hope until Dr. Paul's and Dr. Patrick's LifeCall program", she exclaimed.

Betty is an inspiration to anyone who is facing weight and health conditions. Her determination and hard work are providing her with a new outlook on her life. She is a perfect example of how strong faith and support from others are essential to conquer adversity and promote positive changes.

• • • • •

My name is Ken Rice. I am a 62 yr old man that had never had chiropractic care.

In 2009 I had a total hip replacement which was the result of osteoarthritis. At this time I was given a prescription of Meloxican for the arthritis. Six months later I started having pain in my neck. I went to my primary care and he referred me to a spine surgeon. I was sent for a cat scan with dye. The result came back that I would need to have a procedure to put cadaver bones in my neck due to the osteoarthritis. After praying about my situation I decided to hold off on the surgery, at which time they recommended I stay on the Meloxican. I was also on blood pressure meds and had been for quite some time. I am a local beekeeper in Fairfield, Ohio. In the summer of 2012 it was time to extract honey.

I was out on one of the farms pulling boxes off the hives that were full of honey. Each box weighs approx. 65-70 lbs. I must have turned the wrong way and a pain shot across my lower back and down my left leg. I thought I strained something and with some rest, it would be ok. The pain didn't go away. So I went to my primary care physician. They took x-rays and sent me to a neurosurgeon. He said I had a herniated disc, and we would try epidural injections. I went thru a series of those with little or no results. All the time remaining in almost unbearable pain. I couldn't stand walk or lie down without the pain. I was desperate for some relief and I didn't know where to turn.

A wonderful friend that goes to our church (Geneva Lewis) begged me to go see Dr. Patrick Baker. This was approx. 2 months after

I had injured my back. I made the appointment. The day of the appointment I could barely walk in the office. I was slumped over and the pain was obvious on my face. Dr Bakers staff greeted me and took me right back and did x-rays and scanned my back. The scan showed my neck and left lower back were severe. I waited in the Dr's office and Dr. walked in and said Mr. Rice, We are going to help you. They had me hang over a machine as long as I could. He adjusted me and when I got up off that table I was standing straight and my pain was decreased by 40%. I could not believe what one visit did for my pain. With every visit my back continued to improve until I was pain free. We are still working on my neck, which was more severe than my back. I have so much confidence in Dr Baker and his amazing staff that I know we will get my neck pain free also.

My wife Carol and I took a 30 day challenge that the Fairfield office offered. It was literally a life changing experience for us. We were to use recipes from the Maximized Living nutritional plans, a book offered at Dr Patrick Baker's office. We weighed in on a machine that told your weight, body fat percentage, and muscle mass. After the weigh in, we started our 30 day challenge. The recipes in the book I will have to say are absolutely delicious. We started every morning with a protein shake which was a scoop of Maximized Living Protein powder. That is added to 1 cup of almond milk. To that I would add fresh Kale, fresh strawberries, fresh pineapple, a few almonds. The book is a wealth of knowledge for nutritional values on various things. For example, you would need to eat 20 bowls of oatmeal to equal the nutritional value of I bowl of Kale. I put the fresh kale in the protein shake and when you blend it up you don't even taste the kale. After a couple weeks we realized this was a life style change we could live with. We both work, so what makes it nice is any of the recipes can be done in 20 minutes or less. The recipes literally explode with flavor. After 30 days we weighed in. I lost 14.2 lbs. and reduced my body fat by 2.8%.

My wife did even better reducing her body fat by 3.6%. An added amazing fact is that both my wife and I are off all prescription meds.

Including blood pressure, arthritis meds, acid reflux meds, and cholesterol meds, just as a side note. The acid reflux was caused by the extended use of arthritis medications. It is now 61/2 weeks and I am down 20lbs. and my wife Carol is doing well. We monitor our blood pressure every morning just to keep tabs. So far both are at or slightly below normal with no meds.

We are at a point in our lives that we are living a much healthier life because of the total program Dr. Patrick baker and his amazing staff offer for everyone. It's not a diet. It's keeping your spine in alignment and discovering a nutritional plan you can follow and enjoy the rest of your life.

I thank God for directing our path to Dr. Patrick Baker and his staff. Dr. Baker and his staff truly care about a person's quality of life. My wife and I are living proof.

God Bless.

- **Ken Rice**

Other Books by Dr. Paul Baker and Dr. Patrick Baker

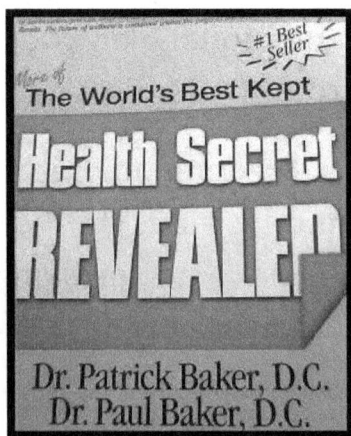

Order your copies on-line at
www.doctorspaulandpatrick.com

www.ingramcontent.com/pod-product-compliance
Lightning Source LLC
Chambersburg PA
CBHW060452290526
45791CB00001B/80